D0901234

MEMORY MAKEOVER

HOW TO PREVENT ALZHEIMER'S AND REVERSE COGNITIVE DECLINE THE NATURAL WAY

DR. WES YOUNGBERG

Find us on the web at *winwellness.org and dryoungberg.com*

ISBN Paperback: 978-0-9824979-1-3

Editors: John B. Youngberg, EdD, Professor Emeritus, Andrews University; Beverly Boyson Youngberg, MAT; Candice Hollingsead, PhD; Conna Bond, JD

Design and typesetting: Donna Cunningham of BeauxArts.Design

PLEASE NOTE: This book contains stories and case studies involving patients the author and his colleagues have worked with in the past. Their names and identities have been changed to protect their privacy and in the interest of confidentiality. The information in this book is for educational purposes only. It is designed to help you make informed decisions about your health, but is not intended to be a substitute for professional medical advice. Always consult your healthcare provider to determine the appropriateness of the information for your own situation. If you need specific advice, seek help from a medical professional who is knowledgeable in that area. The author and publisher specifically disclaim all responsibility for any liability, loss, or risk, personal or otherwise, which is incurred as a consequence, directly or indirectly, of the use and application of any of the contents of this book.

CONTENTS

ABOUT THE AUTHOR

MY SON, WES YOUNGBERG, was born on August 1, 1960, in Temuco, Chile, in South America where my wife Bonnie and I were serving as missionaries. When Bonnie was five months pregnant, she almost lost Wes. In tears, she prayed, "Lord, I love my baby! Save my baby!" God did not allow His plans for healing to the nations to be curtailed, and by divine providence Wes's life was spared.

When Wes was 10, Bonnie fell ill in Bolivia with a glioblastoma. After returning to the U.S., she passed to her rest in 1971. This awakened in Wes a passion to learn how to prevent such tragedies in himself and others.

After earning his bachelor's degree in Health and Physical Education, Wes enrolled at Loma Linda University where he earned a Master of Public Health in Nutrition and a Doctor of Public Health specializing in Clinical Preventive Care. He worked for 14 years as a medical missionary on the island of Guam where he headed the governor's task force for treating and preventing diabetes. When the education of his children called for a return stateside, by vote of the legislature the governor of Guam presented Wes with the Ancient Order of the Chamarri Award—the highest honor the government of Guam grants to any non-Guamanian.

Expanding his practice in 2016, Wes trained and earned certification in the Bredesen Protocol with Dr. Dale E. Bredesen, MD, of the University of California, Los

Angeles, Department of Alzheimer's Research and author of the book *The End of Alzheimer's*.

Together, Wes and I climbed Mt. Tunari, the highest mountain in the Central Bolivian Andes (elevation 17,060 feet)—28 years after failing our initial attempt. (If you have failed in your health initiatives, there are second chances!) As we rose above the surrounding peaks one step at a time, our bodies panted from oxygen deprivation. Nonetheless, when we arrived at the summit, Wes—in true form—did a handstand on the high point.

Today, Wes is helping hundreds of people scale heights and achieve optimal health and wellness. He's also helping them avoid the dangerous precipices of Alzheimer's Disease and cognitive decline. More than half of Wes's patients request guidance regarding Alzheimer's and other forms of cognitive decline. Many are referred by Dr. Bredesen and other neurologists.

In addition to serving as an assistant clinical professor for the Loma Linda University Schools of Medicine and Public Health, Wes is a certified nutrition specialist and a founding director and fellow of the American College of Lifestyle Medicine. He is the author of *Goodbye Diabetes* and *Hello Healthy* as well as the co-author of a series of books entitled *Getting Started, Pressing Forward,* and *Finishing Strong.* Those books examine 21 essential strategies for preventing disease and enjoying optimal wellness. They expand on the foundational principles necessary for optimizing brain wellness and are illustrated by 1,300 PowerPoint slides for small group and public presentation.

Memory Makeover—How to Prevent Alzheimer's and Reverse Cognitive Decline the Natural Way is the fourth in that series. *Jesus—Who Is He?* is the fifth and is written by myself and my wife Millie Youngberg. We are both professors emeriti of Andrews University.

Together, this five-book series comprises the *WIN! Wellness—On The Path To Health and Healing* program, most of which has been translated into 31 languages and used on 6 continents. That program comprehensively addresses multiple links in the healing chain that bring health and healing to tens of thousands of people globally.

Wes and his wife Betsy have three children—Dakota, Madie, and Katie. He currently treats patients at the Youngberg Lifestyle Medicine Clinic in Temecula, California. He also consults with patients by phone or Skype to help reduce their travel expenses. You may visit his website at www.dryoungberg.com or call 951-676-9922 to schedule a consultation.

John Youngberg, EdD
Co-Author, WIN! Wellness

INTRODUCTION

It was the best of times, it was the worst of times,
it was the age of wisdom, it was the age of foolishness,
it was the epoch of belief, it was the epoch of incredulity,
it was the season of light, it was the season of darkness,
it was the spring of hope, it was the winter of despair.

Charles Dickens
A Tale of Two Cities

MOST ARE FAMILIAR with the opening lines from Charles Dickens' *A Tale of Two Cities*. If I didn't know better, I'd think that passage was a brilliant introduction to the current state and practice of preventing and treating Alzheimer's. Dickens believed that renewal and transformation is possible at personal and societal levels. I believe it is also possible with regard to our physical and mental health.

If he were alive today, Dickens might observe that segments of our modern medical system are struggling to defend their reluctance to accept the hundreds of studies that point towards revolution in the art and practice of medicine. This revolution seeks to surge beyond despair and suffering towards a future full of joy and hope.

That is, in fact, what this book is all about. It is a guide to help you move past the current mindset that Alzheimer's is still shrouded in mystery without any viable solutions.

Knowledge of the science and underlying triggers of cognitive decline have placed us in an unparalleled age of wisdom, and yet relatively few of us in the healing professions have been willing to integrate this newfound wisdom into our day-to-day patient care. Most of us are so grounded in convention that strategies inconsistent with traditional standards of care are considered foolish. Some of us are cynical of new information, discrediting its merits and leaving our patients in darkness.

Then again, others of us are embracing "new light" as we see evidence of its benefits to our patients. Personally, I have witnessed patients emerge from the *winter of despair* and experience the *spring of hope*. All they need is guidance and direction.

Few patients or families put significant effort into slowing, stopping, or even reversing cognitive decline when little hope or direction is given during their diagnostic consultations. But how many might, with a little encouragement, embrace the potential for healing provided by a comprehensive and individualized wellness protocol?

As Dickens points out, major change rarely occurs without a conflict that requires a revolutionary overthrow of outdated yet firmly held beliefs. Revolutionary thought ultimately allows for a rebirth of sorts; it brings with it a transformation that was previously thought impossible. If we accept the outdated belief that nothing can be done about Alzheimer's, then of course we are unlikely to put forth much effort into altering its course in our lives or the lives of those we love.

If we want to get better, then clearly our first step is to *reject* the notion that getting better is impossible. To succeed and get past the entrenched boundaries of hopelessness, we must, at least in our own minds, overthrow the idea that cognitive decline can't be reversed.

Accomplishing this can be compared to planting seeds in good soil. There is no harvest unless first the seeds are planted. The next steps require proper nourishment from water, minerals from the soil, and sunshine from above. There are, in fact, many other environmental factors and conditions that influence healthy growth. Growth resulting from proper nourishment is analogous to embracing and applying all the knowledge currently available in published, peer-reviewed scientific literature that represents change that is necessary for actualization, transformation, and healing to occur—a changing of the guard, so to speak.

After 30 years of clinical experience using lifestyle medicine and functional nutrition strategies in the prevention, treatment, and reversal of chronic diseases like diabetes, heart disease, depression, anxiety, chronic kidney disease, neuropathies, autoimmune disease, gastrointestinal/digestive ailments, hormonal imbalances, inflammatory challenges, and so forth, I've learned that each and every chronic disease and its multiple risk factors has an effect on the brain and cognitive function. If we want to avoid Alzheimer's, we must first optimally manage, step-by-step, the risk factors associated with those chronic diseases.

This book is not intended to provide all the answers. I have written multiple books that more fully expand on the natural strategies for reversing health risks. This book is designed as a guide on applying those remedies within the context of Alzheimer's and mild cognitive impairment. I have largely chosen to use stories and case studies from my own clinic as well as from various colleagues. Reading how others worked through each of their health challenges will give you an understanding of how to get started and, most importantly, a willingness to see it through.

CHAPTER 1

DEFINITION OF ALZHEIMER'S

ALZHEIMER'S DISEASE IS A FORM OF DEMENTIA, a decline in mental ability severe enough to interfere with the activities of daily living. Alzheimer's is by far the most common form of dementia, accounting for 80 percent of all cases.[1] There are three primary levels of cognitive decline: 1) subjective cognitive decline, 2) mild cognitive decline, and 3) Alzheimer's Disease ranging from mild to moderate and ultimately to severe loss of cognitive function.

The patient stories described in this book will further define and discuss each level of cognitive decline. The stories will also clearly demonstrate how a personalized wellness protocol, based on extensive lab testing and risk factor analysis, can bring about improvements in brain health for individuals at every stage of cognitive decline. I have personally seen hundreds of patients, ranging from very mild cognitive concerns to severe Alzheimer's dementia, improve their cognitive function and brain health. I'd love to include many of them in this "how to" guidebook, but that will have to wait for a future edition. In the case studies I'm including in this edition, I have incorporated information and explanations that will help you better understand how to initiate and succeed in developing your own personalized wellness protocol.

THREE GOALS OF TREATMENT

When I see new patients concerned about their memory or changes in cognition, I tell them we have three goals. The first goal is to slow the progression of cognitive decline. The second is to stop the progression. The third is to reverse as many aspects of cognitive decline as possible.

Overall, the main goal is to become more functional in the tasks of daily living. I explain to them that, while short-term memory is very important, it is not nearly as important as being able to independently dress, shower, wash and comb their hair, and recognize family members.

I then candidly discuss with them where their cognitive decline is most likely headed. Unless they have lived with a parent who experienced years of persistent decline, most have very little understanding of what is on their horizon, unless the underlying risk factors are identified and effectively addressed.

It's possible that your cognitive decline may be so mild that only you notice its effects. In contrast, your spouse or a parent's cognitive decline may be so severe they now require assistance in nearly all their daily activities—unable to effectively communicate, tell time, know where or who they are, or remember how to dress, eat, bathe, and even use the toilet.

While there is no guarantee that healing at any level will take place, the majority of my patients who have followed their personalized wellness protocol for at least six months have been able to stop the progression of dementia and also experience at least some aspect of reversal of cognitive decline. I have experienced a few notable exceptions, including a case where a middle-aged man brought his lovely wife to see me. She was only 49 when first diagnosed with Alzheimer's. Early onset Alzheimer's that starts before age 65 is very rare, representing only five percent of cases; clearly, her situation was very unusual. Her dementia had progressed rapidly, and now three years later she was experiencing significant challenges with the activities of daily living.

Her husband had witnessed dramatic improvements in a friend who had worked with me on a monthly basis through phone consultations. Eagerly, he initiated the comprehensive testing for his wife and carefully oversaw the personalized wellness protocol we developed for her over time. After 18 months of applying the best strategies currently available in functional and lifestyle medicine, it was clear that his relatively young wife's dementia was not only unusual, but also relentless. While her personalized wellness protocol had done wonders for many of her health risk factors, it had not come in time or effectively stopped her progression into severe Alzheimer's. While very disappointed, her husband found great peace in the fact that he had done everything possible for his wife of more than 30 years.

The occasional case like that one motivates me to never stop learning, to continually apply new scientific findings to my clinical protocols, and to do all I can to find the missing pieces in each patient's health puzzle. Each patient presents with unique genetic, environmental, and lifestyle-related risk factors. Our job as a doctor and patient team is to do our homework and put our best effort towards fixing every risk factor we discover. As I see more and more patients experience improvements in cognitive function, I am reminded over and over that, regardless of the stage of cognitive decline, there is always hope.

ALZHEIMER'S DISEASE RISK FACTORS

Out of 7 million people in the United States who currently have dementia, a full 5.4 million have Alzheimer's. Worldwide, more than 30 million people suffer from Alzheimer's. Researchers estimate that, over the next 30 years, 160 million individuals will be living with Alzheimer's. Of the 326 million people now alive in the United States, 45 million will eventually be diagnosed with Alzheimer's in our lifetime. Amazingly, that number might be four times larger, but most of us who are at risk will die prematurely from heart disease, diabetes, cancer, and other chronic illnesses before falling victim to Alzheimer's Disease.[2]

The spotlight on the magnitude of Alzheimer's has increased, with a recent epidemiological report clarifying that Alzheimer's is now the third leading cause of death in the United States.[3] A woman's chance of developing Alzheimer's is now greater than her chance of developing breast cancer.[4] As of 2015, dementia and Alzheimer's are now reported to be the number one cause of death for women in the United Kingdom.

Overall, it is also the most common cause of death in men and women who are older than 80 years.[5] Public Health England reports that life expectancy has increased to 79.5 years for men who can expect to live the last fifth of their life in poor health. Women now live even longer, to an average of 83.1 years, but they can expect to spend "nearly a quarter of their lives in ill-health."[6]

Unless there is a drastic change in our understanding of what factors contribute to Alzheimer's, what the multiple underlying triggers are, and what we can do to prevent this disease, we will all be at risk of becoming just another statistic. Those of us who survive into our mid 80s have nearly a 50 percent chance of developing Alzheimer's.

On a personal level, the questions we should be asking are: Am I at risk? Are the ones I love at risk? As I write this, I'm 59 years old; within another 10 years, 1 out of 5 people my age or older will have Alzheimer's. The risk grows each year. By the time I reach 85 years of age, 40 to 50 percent of us will have Alzheimer's—unless, of course, we embrace the age of wisdom, the season of light, and the spring of hope.

In this book, I share actual stories and case studies of people just like you and me who had their hopes and dreams shattered by a dreaded diagnosis, yet were able to experience healing. Through these stories, I explain the process they went through to accomplish their goals.

There are so many stories I could tell, but that would require a much larger book. Let's start this journey with the wonderful love story of Mary and John.

CHAPTER 2

Mary and John
Case Study

During a recent phone consultation with John, I commiserated with him about the cost of specialized clinical care for his wife, Mary, who had been diagnosed with advanced Alzheimer's Disease five years earlier. He explained that the disease had left her unable to function in daily life. Her attempts to communicate with family members were unintelligible "jibber jabber." She no longer smiled, nor was she able to show normal emotions. She frequently became agitated and uncontrollable.

Love Story

The neurologist who had diagnosed Mary with Alzheimer's in 2014 had initially prescribed Aricept. He had her discontinue it because there was no noticeable benefit and it made her more aggressive. He then prescribed Memantine 10 mg. That medication didn't produce any benefit either, but with no better options and because it didn't cause aggressiveness or other side effects, it was continued and gradually increased. Mary's mental function continued to steadily decline.

By 2015, at the age of 66, Mary was experiencing advanced symptoms of Sundown Syndrome. Every evening about an hour or two before sundown, Mary would become increasingly agitated and confused. She would hallucinate that dead relatives were in her room talking with her and would pack her suitcase. John would spend the rest of the evening, often up to four hours, trying to calm his wife down and keep her from walking out the front door. She wanted to "go home and be with my mother," even though Mary's mother had been dead for decades. Every morning for the next three-and-a-half years, John lovingly took the time to unpack all of Mary's bags and carefully reorganize her clothes in her closet and dressers.

TESTING FOR COGNITIVE IMPAIRMENT

Early in 2018, Mary's neurologist tested her cognitive abilities with the 30-point Montreal Cognitive Assessment (MoCA) test. Normal cognition allows patients to score at least 27 out of the 30 points on the test. Scoring 18 to 26 points is considered indicative of mild cognitive impairment. Scoring 11 to 17 points indicates mild dementia and is associated with the early stage of Alzheimer's. A MoCA score of 6 to 10 suggests moderate dementia and a more progressive form of Alzheimer's. But scores of less than 6 are consistent with severe dementia and very advanced Alzheimer's.

"So Sorry"

John was stunned and demoralized when Mary's neurologist explained to him that his wife of 40 years hadn't even scored one point on the 30-point MOCA test. Mary's score was zero. The doctor then repeated the three words he had said so often to other patients. "I'm so sorry," he said, putting his hand on John's shoulder. He then suggested that John seriously should consider placing his wife in a residential memory care certified nursing home. He took John aside and suggested that the physical and emotional demands of continuing to care for Mary at home would very likely place him at great personal health risk and ultimately destroy his own health prematurely.

Lost Soul—Scared and Confused

The doctor went on to explain that caring for an advanced Alzheimer's patient isn't like caring for a loved one who needs 24-hour support for three to six months until they get better.

"Even though Mary has advanced Alzheimer's," he said, "she is physically fit and could easily live another 10 years. But when patients like her progress this far into dementia, there is no turning back. Physically, they live on for many years, but mentally they are 'lost souls' who are scared and confused. They often don't know where they are or why they don't recognize anyone. They get to the point where they don't even know who they are themselves.

"It is a terrifying process for the patient," the doctor continued. "The best we can do is to get them the help they need, providing the hour by hour assistance necessary for them to make it through the day. You can visit her every day at the assisted living home. This way you can be sure to get the sleep *you* need to stay healthy and not get burned out by the constant hour-by-hour attention required to care for Mary."

FOR BETTER OR WORSE

John couldn't believe it had come to this. He and Mary had frequently talked about growing old together and relishing their golden years after retirement. Traveling together and enjoying their grandchildren had been their anticipated reward after four decades of hard work. But now, all their dreams seemed to be like a beautiful vase of flowers that had just slipped through their fingers and shattered on the floor. John couldn't even think of how to respond. As the doctor escorted him and Mary back to the waiting room, John took a deep breath and said that he would make some phone calls.

After calling his adult children, John made phone calls to a few assisted living facilities. Not only could he not bear the thought of moving Mary out of their home, but he also John was shocked at the expense of placing Mary into a residential memory care facility. Each place he called explained that even the basic level of care required well over $100,000 each year.

At that point, John decided that he was going to invest his energy in figuring out the actual causes of Mary's cognitive decline. It seemed logical to him that there had to be one or more factors that were contributing to his wife's deteriorating mental status. If he could just find out what those factors were and get them treated, maybe Mary's cognitive function would gradually improve.

RESEARCHING ON THE INTERNET

Not willing to give up quite yet, he decided to do some research on the Internet. He was overwhelmed by multiple reports recommending countless conflicting ideas, including special exercises, brainteaser games, low-fat diets, high-fat diets, plant-based diets, and meat-based paleo diets. Most confusing were the hundreds of nutritional supplements that were purported to benefit the brain. Some of the information looked very interesting, some simply looked "too good to be true," and others looked shady at best.

He was surprised, however, to find many studies published in reputable scientific journals suggesting there were factors that should at least be evaluated as potential causes of Alzheimer's. If each risk factor were properly tested for and appropriately treated, Mary could potentially stop or even reverse some of her symptoms of cognitive decline.

John also took the time to read several books, including *The End of Alzheimer's* by Dr. Dale Bredesen. Because all the research was overwhelming, he realized that he desperately needed expert guidance in figuring out how to apply what he was learning to Mary's situation. He made some notes and then wrote out a list of questions to take to Mary's neurologist.

CARING NEUROLOGIST

John was grateful that their neurologist was kind and willing to discuss his questions.

"Is it reasonable for me to think that optimizing Mary's diet, getting her to start exercising, and then testing for and treating any known 'potential Alzheimer's risk factor' could actually help stop Mary's mental decline or, better yet, start healing her brain?"

The neurologist pondered John's question for a moment. He didn't want to give any false hope. He explained that the field of neurology currently offers no cure or solution for Alzheimer's Disease. He continued to explain that there are population-based studies suggesting benefits from various lifestyle factors, including diet and exercise, but there is currently no official endorsement of any protocol that would effectively slow or reverse symptoms of cognitive decline.

Of course, there would be no harm in promoting a better diet for Mary, especially since she was diabetic. In addition, a daily exercise routine would be good for Mary's anxiety and depression. So why not? Sure! It would be worth the effort.

REPORTS ON COGNITIVE DECLINE REVERSAL

Recognizing that John was willing to do anything and everything to help his wife, the neurologist suggested to John something he had not mentioned to any other patient. In the latter part of 2017, he had attended a presentation I had given at the annual conference of the American College of Lifestyle Medicine. There, I had presented on the work of Dr. Dale Bredesen, a research neurologist and professor at University of California, Los Angeles (UCLA) School of Medicine.

Dr. Bredesen had published a paper in 2014 in the journal *Aging*.[7] In this paper he had described how 9 out of 10 patients with cognitive impairment and/or early forms of Alzheimer's had reversed the functional signs and symptoms of cognitive decline in less than a year's time by following a comprehensive wellness protocol. Since Dr.

Bredesen was the first to publish papers on the effectiveness of simultaneously combining multiple strategies into one comprehensive functional protocol, many of us who specialize in this clinical approach refer to it as the "Bredesen Protocol."

This protocol essentially seeks to address any and all known potential risk factors for Alzheimer's. It does so by broadly testing for as many risk factors as possible and then seeking not just to normalize but to optimize them. Mary's neurologist had spoken with me after my presentation, showing great interest in this revolutionary concept. We discussed the very controversial aspect of even suggesting that *reversal* of cognitive decline was possible.

The neurologist knew that simply telling all his Alzheimer's patients to start following this protocol would be met by criticism and frustration from other doctors. Ultimately, criticism would also come from his patients if they were only looking for a simple fix and were unwilling to change their lifestyle at the level required by the protocol.

He had cautiously decided to wait for a patient who had a spouse or family member who was clearly ready for such advice and also willing to put forth the time and effort needed to give it an honest chance of working. And here now was John, asking whether there was anything else he could do to keep the love of his life home with him as long as possible.

Willing to take the risk, Mary's neurologist told John about my talk at the American College of Lifestyle Medicine. He told him about the nine patients who had, in dramatic fashion, reversed their cognitive decline. He cautioned John not to expect a reversal in Mary's condition, especially because of her advanced case of Alzheimer's. But, he said, "There's nothing to lose and everything to gain from at least trying. Why not give it a shot, and even if it doesn't help much, it just might help some."

Given the complexity of Mary's medical challenges, the neurologist suggested that John set up a series of phone consultations with me. For the first time in years, John had something to hang his hopes on. Walking out of the neurology clinic that day with Mary holding onto his arm, John started to smile. He remembered the challenges Henry Ford had endured while revolutionizing the automobile industry. Nearly everyone had told Henry Ford, "It can't be done."

In response, Ford quipped, "Whether you think you can, or think you can't, you're right!"

As John and Mary drove home that day, John purposed in his heart that he would do everything he could for Mary. He wasn't going to just sit back and let Alzheimer's take his wonderful wife of 40 years away from him—not without a fight! Another smile creased his face; this time it was faint, but confident. He looked over at Mary who was watching him with those big, trusting eyes. Mary knew she was safe with John and couldn't help but smile back.

As they came to stop in front of their house, John decided that his only hope was to act. After Mary was settled in her favorite chair, John made his first phone call to our clinic. Even though the couple lived in the Eastern United States, he was more than willing to fly with Mary to San Diego and spend as much time as needed to get Mary tested and started on the protocol. However, he was pleased to discover that he could get all the labs done in his own city, and all the consultations could be done by either phone or Skype.

CHAPTER 3

FORMULA FOR HOPE

DAY ONE: FIRST CONSULTATION

My first consultation with John was in late July of 2018. During the initial consultation, my goal was to listen intently and learn as much as I could from him about Mary's current condition and the progression of symptoms over the last years and decades.

There is a principle of good medicine first noted by the famous doctor Sir William Osler, one of the first chiefs of medicine at Johns Hopkins Hospital and School of Medicine. "Listen to your patient," he admonished. "He is telling you the diagnosis."

I actually said to John, "If I listen to you patiently and for a long enough time, you will tell me exactly what we need to do in order to start Mary on her path to health and healing."

For that first phone consult, I spent a full hour listening, at times asking questions and then listening some more. The next steps were to properly assess risk and then to explain how each risk factor could be effectively addressed.

This is the very process that gives hope. Being told that there is *nothing* that can be done to alter the course of cognitive decline is not only bad medicine, but it also destroys hope! It destroys the most important ingredient of the healing process. But John was fortunate enough to have a neurologist who wasn't willing to destroy his hope for Mary's improvement.

DOCUMENTING BASELINE SYMPTOMS AND RISKS

As we proceeded, it was important to document Mary's current symptoms so we could objectively evaluate the success or failure of my recommendations. John outlined for me a long list of Mary's symptoms: putting clothes on backward since early 2017; inability to bathe herself since 2016; inability to fix food for herself but capacity to use eating utensils without support; inability to spread peanut butter on bread; putting her left shoe on her right foot; inability to have a conversation with family members; memories consistent with when she was 8 or 9 years old; inability to converse in a way that made sense.

CONSENSUS-BASED MEDIOCRITY VS. CUTTING-EDGE PROTOCOLS

After John reviewed Mary's medical history and current symptoms with me, I too cautioned John regarding his expectations. However, I also told him there is always hope. No one, especially doctors, should say that there is no hope—it's simply not true! There is always hope when there is a willingness to go beyond the mediocrity of normative- and consensus-based protocols. Relying on consensus-based medical protocols is essentially rejecting more advanced, cutting-edge medical strategies that typically take decades to gain mainstream acceptance.

I learned long ago that trying to justify what I do clinically to skeptical health professionals is a poor use of my time. Convincing others against their will simply takes too much time away from actually helping patients who are eager to prevent or reverse disease. I'd much rather spend my time helping patients like Mary who are ready to try a different treatment than to waste my time debating doctors who haven't read the studies for themselves.

John and Mary had several things going for them. They had a caring and open-minded neurologist, and I could tell that John was not going to "go silently into the night." He was going to fight for Mary—and keep fighting for her no matter what. He was not going to let anyone smooth talk him into losing hope.

When preparing for the initial testing phase, I tell patients and their spouses or supporting health partners that our goal is to find as many active risk factors as possible. They often look at me quizzically as if to say, "I don't want to discover I have any additional health problems."

To this I say, "If we don't find any risk factors, our ability to improve your brain health is greatly limited. The more risk factors we find and fix, the greater your chances of significant reversal of cognitive decline."

Once they understand this, they are eager to discover new risk factors and do whatever it takes to optimize each one.

Because the protocol is so comprehensive in its approach to numerous risk factors, it takes time to address them properly. For this reason, I typically schedule patients for a full-hour consultation once a month until we properly address every risk factor discovered through the comprehensive testing protocol.

After an average of three months on the full protocol, we retest. This time we test only labs that needed to improve. If the new lab is now in the optimal range, we simply maintain the current protocol used to make the improvement. If necessary, we adjust the protocol in order to get further improvement.

It generally takes 6 to 12 months before we reach a maintenance phase, at which point we only need to meet every 3 months for a while, and then every 6 months to a year thereafter.

ASSESSING MARY'S RISK FACTORS

In mid-August, just three weeks after our initial consultation, we began addressing each specific risk factor revealed by the comprehensive lab testing Mary completed at a lab near her home. Broad testing allows discovery of risk factors patients have had for many years but didn't know about. It's sad, but true. We all have risk factors for Alzheimer's, but few of us know which risk factors we carry. That is because no one has bothered to check them.

It's crazy to think that we could have prevented our health problem but never thought of checking our risk factors when we were much younger. It would be wise to do this same comprehensive testing in our early 40s or even earlier. This would give us a 20- to 30-year running start in catching many risk factors and properly treating them before they have a chance of causing cognitive decline or Alzheimer's.

CHAPTER 4

NEW PERSPECTIVE ON DEMENTIA

AFTER YEARS OF SEEING THE EBB and tide of dementia symptoms in many patients, my perspective on what dementia really is has changed. Patient caregivers and family members often asked me why some days their spouse or parent did so much better than normal, and then other days their cognitive function was especially poor. It has long been believed that dementia is simply a progressive condition that happens to us because of uncontrollable genetic factors. But it became increasingly clear to me that my patients' symptoms were often related to something that had changed fairly recently.

Over time, I began to realize that dementia symptoms were caused by being under the influence of something or multiple things that collectively caused dementogenic symptoms within minutes to hours after exposure. In other words, dementia symptoms can be turned up or down, on or off, and activated or deactivated based on the sum total of exposome.

Our exposome includes everything we are exposed to from our environment—everything we do, everything we eat, everything we drink, everything we say, hear, think, and dwell on. It includes everything in our lives. This is precisely why each of us must evaluate how our brain is uniquely at risk from various exposomal factors that literally change the way our genes work.

Based on these observations, I tend to think of dementia as a temporary cognitive impairment associated with recent exposures to one or more dementogens that collectively cross a threshold level, leading to decreased functionality in judgement, communication, organization, and the normal functions of daily living. If this is accurate, then our first responsibility is to discover as many of these dementogens as possible and then do our very best to remove them from our lives. Our second responsibility is to discover as many of the factors that help neutralize or even reverse the dementogenic effects of our past and current exposures.

In Mary's case, we found many risk factors that had previously gone unnoticed. John was prepared for this. As I pointed out more and more risk factors that we would be seeking to optimize, John became increasingly hopeful. He knew that uncovering more risk factors meant more effective treatments for the underlying triggers of Mary's Alzheimer's. I'll examine those risk factors in the rest of the book.

ELEVATED HOMOCYSTEINE – A NEUROTOXIN

Mary's homocysteine level was 15—very high. Many studies clearly show that elevated homocysteine acts as a neurotoxin and is associated with premature death of memory cells in our brain's hippocampus. In fact, a high homocysteine more than triples the risk of developing Alzheimer's.

We immediately started Mary on therapeutic levels of three key supplemental nutrients: vitamin B12 as methyl-cobalamin, vitamin B9 as methyl folate, and vitamin B6 as pyridoxal 5 phosphate. The dose required to optimize homocysteine levels differs among patients and therefore must be individualized based on multiple factors.

DHEA, Pregnenolone and Thyroid— Neuroprotective Hormones

Initial testing revealed that Mary had suboptimal levels of multiple hormones that help protect the brain and memory cells. In particular, she was low in DHEA sulfate, an adrenal hormone. She was also low in pregnenolone, a master hormone often referred to as the "memory hormone." Right away, we initiated a conservative dose with breakfast and lunch.

We also noticed that, while Mary's thyroid profile was technically within the normal statistical range, it was clearly not in the optimal range. Both of her thyroid hormones—the Free T4 and the Free T3—were at the bottom of the reference range. Many doctors think this is acceptable. Being in the low normal range meant that Mary's thyroid hormones were actually lower than the levels of more than 90 percent of the population!

Additionally, Mary had significantly elevated antibodies in her blood that were attacking her thyroid gland. In fact, they were 500 percent higher than the maximum level considered to be normal. This test indicated that we needed to incorporate strategies to effectively address Mary's newly discovered autoimmune condition. Fortunately, there are many ways to calm autoimmunity. This includes optimizing hormones, as demonstrated by the Cleveland Clinic and others.[8] [9]

AUTOIMMUNE RISK

At this point, I started educating John about treating the underlying causes of autoimmunity. I also suggested ways to address them with Mary's neurologist at their next visit. Proper thyroid function is so critical to brain function that hypothyroidism (low thyroid levels or function) can cause cognitive impairment and Alzheimer's symptoms all by itself. John agreed to take all the labs and notes to his next doctor visit and request that Mary be started on a low dose of thyroid medication.

After reading my notes discussing the importance of optimizing thyroid function in people with cognitive concerns, Mary's doctor became very supportive and promptly wrote out a prescription for Mary so she could get started on it right away. To make sure the dose was optimal, we scheduled a repeat lab test in 6 weeks.

INFLAMMATION, HSCRP AND BETA AMYLOID BUILDUP

Mary also had a mildly elevated Cardiac CRP (also known as hsCRP), which is a measure of system-wide inflammation. Since inflammation is a major trigger of beta amyloid accumulation in the brain, we initiated natural anti-inflammatory strategies that are known to support cognitive function. This included adding supplemental curcumin and a vegan form of EPA and DHA omega-3 oils. I told John to make sure Mary was getting at least 1,000 mg of DHA daily.

Finally, since 75 percent of Americans are deficient in magnesium, and the goal is to be well into the upper half of the laboratory reference range, I suggested that Mary start Magnesium L-Threonate. This is a form of magnesium that easily crosses the blood brain barrier and helps protect the brain from inflammation and neurotoxins. Diabetics, those with high blood pressure, and anyone at risk of heart disease, depression, anxiety, headaches, etc., benefit greatly from additional supplemental magnesium support.

SUPPLEMENT AVERSION

At this point, some patients say, "I don't want to take supplements. I just want to do this with a whole foods diet."

To this I respond, "A 100 percent whole, plant-based diet is by far the most important and fundamental strategy, and it will be a big part of your health improvement protocol." But the goal is to leave no stone unturned and to do everything that is reasonable.

Remember, if you weren't at risk or didn't have any health problems, you wouldn't need supplemental support, or at least you wouldn't need it as much!
Each risk factor is addressed in the most rational, physiological way and as far upstream as possible. In other words, we treat the risk factor as early as possible in the causal chain of triggering events.

As one example, many of the individual nutrient therapies actually activate the very enzymes that help break down the neurotoxins or the chemicals that trigger inflammation. Using the right nutrients in the right amounts can epigenetically turn your good genes ON and your bad genes OFF. As such, the right nutrients can naturally but effectively inhibit chemicals and enzymes that act on the Amyloid Precursor Protein (APP) to speed up the production of beta amyloid. In other words, the right nutrients at therapeutic levels can slow down the production of excessive beta amyloid plaque.

When produced in excess of the brain's ability to detoxify and remove it, beta amyloid will aggregate into clumps that become neurotoxic, thus damaging memory-containing synapses and neurons. By optimizing your diet and nutrient therapies, you can rev up the expression of genes that help you heal faster, and you can slow down the activation of genes that promote cognitive decline.

The list of potentially beneficial supplemental nutrients and herbs can easily add up to a fairly long list. For this reason, it is important to focus on the supplemental nutrients that specifically match the patient's individual risk profile as determined by their list of diagnosed medical conditions, family history, laboratory tests, and symptoms, etc. The benefit of each nutrient must be re-evaluated periodically based on retesting of the related risk factors.

CHAPTER 5

DOCUMENTING EARLY SUCCESS

SIX WEEKS: PROGRESS INDICATORS

By early September, less than three weeks after John started initiating my recommendations for Mary's personalized wellness protocol, I documented in Mary's clinical notes:

> *Sundowner effect is now somewhat improved. She is less likely now to ask about dead relatives and pack up her bags to go visit them. Now just a casual mention of her mother. Before, her symptoms of Sundown Syndrome were serious and at an intensity of 10/10. As of this consult, her symptoms greatly improved and are now at 2-3/10. Last night, she was able to get ready for bed by herself. Up until recently, Mary had to be coached at every step.*

This improvement in her symptoms and function of daily living had occurred after only six weeks. But John had been working extra hard on implementing an optimal diet and taking Mary on daily walks. This is the most important part of the protocol. Each will be addressed in detail later in this book. Without the foundation of an optimal diet and a regular activity schedule, improvements in cognitive function are unlikely.

DEMENTOGENIC EFFECT OF HIGH AND LOW BLOOD SUGARS

As part of the laboratory review during our September 6 consult, I went over Mary's blood sugar and insulin levels. Mary's fasting blood sugar (glucose) was fine; in fact, it was nearly perfect. But her blood sugars during the 4-hour Glucose Tolerance Test (GTT) told an entirely different story. Her blood sugar levels after the drink were both very high and very low.

Let me explain. After Mary's fasting labs were drawn, the lab technician gave her a carbonated drink that included 75 grams of glucose, which amounts to 300 calories of sugary carbohydrate. This is like drinking an extra sweet Sprite, but it actually only has slightly more sugar than a medium-size soda from McDonald's.

One hour after that drink, Mary's blood sugar shot up to a high of 174 mg/dL. Studies have shown that levels above 150 are strongly associated with cardiovascular disease. The sugar drink raised her blood sugar levels so high that her pancreas had to make excess insulin.

By the second hour of the GTT, Mary's blood sugars had returned to normal, but only because her insulin levels had risen to more than 73 micro Units/mL. This was at least *three times higher* than the more optimal level I recommend, and it provided a big clue as to why Mary was struggling with Alzheimer's.

To make matters worse, the excess insulin eventually caused Mary's blood sugars to come crashing down.

Mary's third- and fourth-hour blood sugars were much lower than they should have been.

Healthy adrenal glands would have produced enough cortisol to gradually release sugar from the liver in order to prevent her hypoglycemic low. We actually measured her adrenal production of cortisol and found that her adrenals were sluggish and very slow to respond. Weak adrenals allowed her blood sugars to crash often, leading to moodiness, fatigue, and even more brain fog than she already had.

MOST COMMON CAUSE OF DEMENTIA

Insulin resistance of the brain makes it hard for the brain cells to access sugar even when blood sugar levels are high. But when blood sugars are low because of hypoglycemic reactions to excess carbohydrates from refined starches and sweets, the brain cells literally start dying. Limiting the brain's access to sugar is like unplugging your computer from its power source while it is saving a large document. Chances are, the document you were saving is now lost.

Likewise, memory synapses and energy-starved brain cells undergo a programmed destruction sequence when "unplugged" from their blood sugar energy source. Unfortunately, as bad as high or low blood sugars are for the brain, a third element exists that creates a "trifecta of risk" and a "perfect storm" that gradually destroys cognitive function.

SWEETS AND EXCESS BETA AMYLOID PRODUCTION IN THE BRAIN

There is another major villain to the brain in this blood sugar roller coaster ride. It has to do with the way excess insulin affects buildup of neurotoxic beta amyloid plaques in the brain. Every time Mary eats her favorite candy or yummy snack, and even every time she overindulges in starches, her blood sugars spike for about an hour, followed by a significant spike of insulin. Excess insulin not only drives the sugar too low, but it also further damages and purges brain cells because it promotes inflammation.

I mentioned earlier that inflammation stimulates the Amyloid Precursor Protein (APP) to speed up the production of beta amyloid. Beta amyloid is a prionic type of protein that actually further amplifies and therefore exponentially speeds up the production of even more beta amyloid. This buildup of amyloid continues to amplify unless significant effort is made to shut it down.

This is one of the reasons many strategies must be followed concurrently to get effective and long-lasting results in reversing cognitive decline. But the "nail in the coffin" from high blood levels of insulin comes from the fact that enzymes in the brain must prioritize the breakdown of high insulin levels in order to prevent even worse damage than can occur from low blood sugars. These enzymes are appropriately called Insulin Degrading Enzymes, also known as IDE's.

INSULIN DEGRADING ENZYME BREAKS UP BETA AMYLOID

Every time Mary eats unhealthfully or enjoys a snack, her insulin levels go up excessively. This requires the IDE's to stop their other job and focus on breaking down the extra insulin. Even if the IDE's keep the insulin spike from lasting too long, there is still a problem. The problem has to do with its other job, which just happens to be breaking down and removing beta amyloid plaques in the brain!

That's right; if the IDE's are allowed to put in a full-day's work as brain detoxification specialists, there is a good chance that the brain's buildup of beta amyloid plaques will start to diminish. But being called off their main job to deal with high insulin levels for one to three hours after every meal or snack leaves little if any time to get any real work done on brain clean-up.

This process is much like building a home next to a river before learning that the area floods every spring. We shouldn't build a house on a known flood plain, and likewise, we shouldn't eat in a way that is all but guaranteed to promote ever-increasing neurotoxic beta amyloid plaques resulting in loss of thousands of memory and other brain cells every day! This eventually leads to impaired cognitive function and, ultimately, Alzheimer's Disease.

Brain Atrophy, Repair & Regrowth of Brain Cells

Researchers have estimated that the average person has about 40 million brains cells (neurons) in their hippocampus[10], which is responsible for organizing short-term memory into long-term memory. The hippocampus also helps us remember where we are and how to get where we are going. It's like a GPS system that keeps us oriented to our environment and keeps us from getting lost or confused. We can safely assume that Mary had lost many millions of brain cells from her hippocampus over the years.

There is actually a fairly long list of poor lifestyle choices and other events and circumstances that can lead to the loss of more than 1,000 hippocampal brain cells every day. Fortunately, neuroscientists have estimated that nearly

1,000 *new* memory cells can be made in the hippocampus of the adult brain each and every day as well.[11]

John's challenge was to help Mary tip the balance toward saving and repairing old brain cells while also making and maintaining new brain cells. Done well and for long enough, Mary could gradually regain and re-establish her previous self.

GOODBYE DIABETES, GOODBYE ALZHEIMER'S

Insulin resistance, with the corresponding excess insulin production, is the most common trigger and driver of dementia over time. This is why many scientists and researchers are referring to Alzheimer's as type 3 diabetes, or more precisely, insulin resistance of the brain.

This concept is so important that I have written a 332-page book on how to reverse insulin resistance. The book is called *Goodbye Diabetes: Preventing and Reversing Diabetes the Natural Way,* and is actually the first resource I recommend to my patients who want to prevent or reverse cognitive decline. I also worked closely with Life & Health Network to film 40 short, seven- to ten-minute videos where I walk viewers through the steps necessary to reverse insulin resistance. This is called the *Diabetes Undone Kit* and includes a full workbook, journal, meal plan, and a plant-based cookbook. Both of these resources are available at www.dryoungberg.com.

I explained to John that getting these resources was not required. The important thing was that they were available to him if he felt he needed more support, examples of how to further optimize the overall protocol, and instructions to build an optimal nutrition and meal plan.

Since John already had the *Goodbye Diabetes* book, I explained to him that each of the 23 chapters sheds additional light on the ways we can reverse insulin resistance and therefore remove the biggest obstacle to repairing Mary's hippocampus and restoring her cognitive abilities. I also encouraged John to watch the *Diabetes Undone* videos on reversing insulin resistance. The *Diabetes Undone* videos and workbook would help John better understand all the factors associated with insulin resistance reversal as well as why walking after every meal would have a powerful impact on Mary's cognitive function.

MOVEMENT MEDICINE

John didn't simply ask Mary whether she wanted to go for a walk. He knew from experience that every time he asked her to go walking with him, she would say NO and stubbornly stick to her guns. No amount of coaxing would change her mind.

But if he said, "Mary, do you want to go shopping?" she would nod, slowly get up, and willingly join him in the car. He would then drive to the mall and they would "shop" from one end of the mall to the other and back. Other times they would go to the grocery store, get a cart for Mary to hold on to, and wander through the produce section and then around the perimeter of the store to the almond milk section, and then back around multiple times. Pretty soon they were walking for about 30 minutes daily. After a while, Mary recognized that she felt better after walks and would even go for walks with John in their neighborhood.

CHAPTER 6

HOPE FOR SUGARHOLICS

Mary was a picky eater and a lifetime sugarholic. She would happily devour any candy, cakes, or pastries within her reach. Not surprisingly, Mary had a history of diabetes and would also experience hypoglycemic reactions because of rapidly dropping blood sugars. I explained to John that both high and low blood sugars are major triggers for dementia.

Since Mary had a tendency to both, we had to prevent the initial spikes of blood sugars after meals and prevent the drops of blood sugar several hours later. To do this, we initiated short walks right after meals and a carefully designed diet that included lots of green leafy and colorful veggies, along with a moderate amount of nuts, seeds, avocados, and olives to help stabilize her blood sugars. We cut out all refined carbohydrates and cold cereals and limited other whole grains.

Fortunately, John was already avoiding the use of any artificial sugars when feeding Mary. It is sad how so many doctors and even national health organizations actually promote the use of artificial sugars. There is plenty of good research documenting its ingestion as being harmful to health and a cause of worsening insulin resistance.

Once again, John didn't ask Mary whether she wanted a smoothie with lots of green leafy veggies blended in with organic blueberries and supplements. John took the time to figure out how to get her to consume it without complaint. John discovered early on that, if left alone, Mary would sneak into the bathroom and flush the smoothie with all the greens, berries, and supplements right down the toilet!

We discussed this and came up with a protocol that would make the smoothie taste good even with all the nasty tasting supplement powders. Since Mary was not able to swallow pills, John would open up each capsule and dump the contents into the smoothie. Adding 2 teaspoons of crushed pineapple made a world of difference in "sweetening the pot" so she would happily drink it all.

SMOOTHIE FOR INGESTING SUPPLEMENTS

Accompany each meal with a 6- to 7-ounce smoothie. Patients are more likely to finish small smoothies than large ones. Blending in supplements makes it easier to get them down, particularly if a patient has trouble swallowing pills.

Ingredients:

4 oz. unsweetened almond milk
1 scoop GlycemaCore (3 flavor options)
2 tsp crushed unsweetened pineapple
1 tbsp old-fashioned peanut or almond butter (optional)
1/3 to 1/2 cup frozen organic blueberries
1/3 to 1/2 scoop Nanogreens

Blend in a Vitamix or similar high-quality blender. In each smoothie, include 1/3 of the daily supplement capsules to be taken with meals for the day. Blend initial ingredients first, then open the supplement capsules and dump the contents into the smoothie and blend again. Make sure all the powder is out of each capsule. Tablets can be crushed into a powder. Gel caps can be cut at one end and the contents squeezed into the smoothie. Finally, blend in 2 teaspoons of crushed, unsweetened pineapple to mask the bitter taste of the powdered supplements. If the color of the mixed ingredients is distracting or distasteful, use a colorful cup, lid, and straw.

This small smoothie makes it easy for patients to consume therapeutic amounts of greens, berries, and supplements without a fuss. success. Mary loved it and, more importantly, finished all of it at each meal, thus ensuring that consumed the many brain-building nutrients.

HEMOGLOBIC A1C TEST AS PREDICTOR OF DEMENTIA RISK

A few years ago, one of my favorite journals, *The New England Journal of Medicine,* published a study showing that elevated blood sugars and A1c levels place people at risk of dementia even if those levels are not high enough to meet the criteria for diabetes.[12] In other words, even mildly elevated blood sugars promote cognitive decline. This is why we must carefully assess how our bodies handle sugar and then fix any problems we find.

To begin with, we tested Mary's Hemoglobin A1c. Ironically, it was perfect at 5.1 percent. Prediabetes doesn't officially begin until the A1c is at least 5.7 percent, and diabetes doesn't begin until the A1c is 6.5 percent or higher. Optimal levels are, in my opinion, 5.1 percent or lower. But in Mary's case the A1c didn't tell us the real story of Mary's significant sugar and insulin problems.

I recommend the A1c test for every patient I see. It is a great test that helps us to understand current and future risk, but it is not nearly as sensitive for determining insulin resistance and spiking of blood sugars after meals.

4-HOUR GLUCOSE TOLERANCE TEST & DEMENTIA RISK

The 4-hour Glucose Tolerance Test is by far the most sensitive and effective lab test for determining any tendency to prediabetes or diabetes. In fact, a 2019 study done by endocrinologists at the City of Hope discovered that the A1c test failed to diagnose an astounding 73 percent of diabetes cases that had been detected by the glucose tolerance test.

Many physicians now primarily use the A1c test to diagnose diabetes. But, according to the study, doing so will result in failure to diagnose nearly three-fourths of patients who actually have diabetes but don't know it because they were not given a glucose tolerance test.

The endocrinologists' recommendation to other clinicians was simple. In addition to the A1c screening test, also order a glucose tolerance test. Yes, the 2-hour Glucose Tolerance Test requires the patient to go to the lab first thing in the morning before breakfast and get a fasting blood sugar. They then drink the 75 grams of Glucola and have their blood sugar checked again 2 hours later. It is indeed a hassle, but quality risk factor assessment is worth the hassle!

If you get a 2-hour Glucose Tolerance Test, make sure your doctor orders the 1-hour blood sugar as well. Many individuals have a perfect fasting blood sugar and a perfect 2-hour blood sugar, but their 1-hour blood sugar is sky high. Even though it is not officially used as a diagnostic measure, the 1-hour blood sugar is the most sensitive indicator of all the blood sugar tests.

That was the case for Mary. Her fasting and 2-hour glucose levels were nearly optimal, but her 1-hour glucose was very high. I also strongly recommend that your doctor order the insulin levels at fasting, 1 hour, and 2 hours into the glucose tolerance test. Insulin levels are even more important than the 1-hour or 2-hour blood sugars.

Not surprisingly, since most doctors are not trained to use the Glucose Tolerance Test, very few feel comfortable ordering it. Even fewer doctors recognize the value of testing insulin or understand how to test for it properly. Consulting with a lifestyle medicine specialist who has experience addressing cognitive decline and Alzheimer's will simplify the process greatly.

CHAPTER 7

Cognitive improvements & Setbacks

Eight Weeks: Reading and Speaking Again in Full Sentences

Since we had so much to address, I met again with John and Mary two weeks later in September. At the beginning of each consultation, I documented whether there were any signs of improvement or worsening of cognitive symptoms. I cautioned John not to over- or understate Mary's current symptoms. If they were worse, our task was to figure out why and then seek to remedy the problem.

John had good news. Here is his report as taken from my notes on that day:

In the last 2 days, Mary has now started to be able to read words on TV and headlines in newspapers and road signs. It has been 3 years since she was able do this. She is now talking in full coherent sentences. It has been over a year and closer to 2 years since this has occurred. This began to happen about 2 days after initiating the newest nutrients discussed at the last consult.

Of course, John had also continued all the previously initiated strategies and made great effort to keep Mary away from all refined foods. He was gradually getting Mary to exercise more.

THREE MONTHS: TRANSFORMATION

On November 1, we met again, and I recorded the following report:

> *Prior to starting the comprehensive wellness protocol, Mary was bed-ridden and slept most of the day. Now she is more active. Mary had not been reading at all for 3 plus years but now is reading often and for the first time in years can identify what time of the day it is. She is now laughing and showing emotion, whereas in the past had no emotion or laughter. She is now aware of where she is. When riding with John in their car, she is aware of how to navigate each turn and even corrects John if he doesn't turn onto the right street or exit. She is now much more interactive, even commenting when watching TV and processing what she is watching. She is regaining the ability to discriminate what is happening or being discussed on the news as good or bad, and as right or wrong.*

A HUSBAND'S COMMITMENT

As I talked further with John, I couldn't help but marvel at his commitment to Mary. We are all human, and it is easy to make excuses as to why we can't get our spouses to consistently follow the program. But I never heard this from John. If there was a challenge, he simply figured out a way around it and made sure that the protocol was followed, no matter what. This was critical, because the next six weeks would be very stressful and push John to the limit. Some would have given up at that point.

FOUR MONTHS: UNEXPECTED SETBACK

On December 19, John and I had our next phone consultation. A perfect storm of unanticipated events had set John and Mary up for unwelcome and very unanticipated setbacks.

While I was enjoying sunny Southern California, John and Mary were experiencing bad winter weather on the East Coast. In a somewhat somber yet resolute tone, John explained to me that, just the day before, Mary had fallen out of bed and broken her leg. To make matters worse, Mary's Sundown Syndrome had returned. Her regression had started two-and-a-half weeks earlier when a winter storm had made it unsafe to continue their daily walks at the high school track and at the nearby soccer field. The roads were icy, causing John to think twice about risking a drive to the mall. Walking at the mall had worked great, but he didn't want to risk a fall from the slippery ice on the parking lot.

RETURN OF SUNDOWN SYNDROME

Without their daily exercise, both John and Mary relaxed their diet. In response to the dreary and gray chill of the winter cold, they started eating more comfort food. Then they cut back the blood sugar balancing smoothie to once a day. Since the supplemental nutrients were added to the smoothie, they inadvertently cut back Mary's intake of the supplements in half. Additionally, Mary had flushed the smoothie with all the supplements down the toilet twice.

John explained, "After one week of being off the second smoothie and not walking regularly, Sundowning came back about 50 percent. This included increased anxiety and delusions that people were waiting for her—primarily relatives that had died years before."

Of interest to me was that, in spite of her partial regression, she did not pack her bags to move back with her mother like she had on most evenings for the past three years. In this regression, she was content to just pack her purse.

UNTIMELY CUT BACK OF NAMENDA

This perfect storm became even more discouraging when, in consultation with their neurologist, Mary's Alzheimer's prescription of Namenda was decreased. Together with their recent failure to follow the comprehensive wellness program, cutting back on the Namenda was ill-timed and led to a noticeable worsening of cognitive symptoms. After this setback, Mary's neurologist increased her Namenda back to the original high dose of 24 mg each day.

LAW OF UNDULATION

In his writings, C.S. Lewis talks about the Principle of Undulation,[13] referring to the peaks and valleys that all humans experience. He writes, "We can easily become confused and discouraged in the valleys of life. And, in the midst of our confusion and discouragement, we are more vulnerable to our own [unhealthy] impulses and to the snares [that so often side track us from doing what is in our best interest]. What can we do in such times? When the clouds of life cast a gray shadow over us, it is especially important to remind ourselves that what we are experiencing is a normal part of life in a fallen world and that in due course the sun will shine again."[14]

For the first four months after our initial consultation, Mary had shown significant and steady improvements in cognitive function. But we all must be prepared for the inevitable ups and downs of life. Health and healing go through phases. It is natural to rejoice during the phase of rejuvenation and steady restoration of health. Likewise, we should expect the inevitable undulations that circumstances and occasional poor choices can bring.

There will be times when, because of accidents, a respiratory illness, travel, or some other life stress, we "fall off the wagon" and find ourselves no longer following the program that had brought so much improvement to our physical and mental health. When this happens, we shouldn't focus on our failure, for it is only temporary. Remember the old adage, "Don't cry over spilled milk." The best response is to acknowledge our mistake, get over it, and immediately get back on track.

GOOD IS THE ENEMY OF BEST

What gets us off track most easily is when we allow a multitude of *good* activities to interfere with our ability to accomplish the *most important* activities of each day. Good things can be the worst enemy of what is best.

Sometimes, a frustrated patient will tell me, "I just can't find the time to exercise daily." I've even been told by some, "I don't have time to take the supplements on my protocol."

The problem is clearly a lack of organization. We must focus on learning how to prioritize how we spend our time. This is done by setting boundaries that protect us from being "nickeled and dimed" by the trivial and nonessential demands on our time. As we learn to say NO to things that are less important, we will have time to do the things that are important.

My patients who most often succeed in reversing at least some aspect of cognitive decline are the ones who effectively set limits and who make room each day to follow every aspect of their personalized

> Sometimes we have to say NO to things we REALLY want to do, in order to say YES to the very best of things.
>
> *Gordon MacDonald*

wellness protocol. Because Mary had advanced Alzheimer's, it was not reasonable to expect her to effectively set limits. For example, Mary loved to eat candy and any form of refined carbohydrates. Simply put, if it was available, she would eat it.

John realized that for Mary to avoid the dementogenic effect of sugar, he needed to be the one to set limits. Likewise, he needed to stick to his guns and not give in to her requests. By making sure that Mary had three well-balanced meals daily, along with her supplemental smoothies, John noticed that Mary became much less likely to request sweets.

Since this principle is so critical, I have given advice to my patients for many years adapted from the following paragraphs originally penned by C.S. Lewis. They speak to the core principles of successfully setting limits and not giving up.

All the contemporary propaganda [for indulgence to our every want] combine to make us feel that the desires we are resisting are so 'natural,' so 'healthy,' and so 'reasonable' that it is almost perverse and abnormal to resist them. Poster after poster, film after film, novel after novel [and commercial after commercial], associate the idea of indulgence with the ideas of health, normality, youth, frankness, and good humor. Now this association is a LIE.

Like all-powerful lies, it is based on a truth – the truth… that [appetite or eating] in itself [apart from the excesses and obsessions that have grown round it] is 'normal' and 'healthy.' The lie consists in the suggestion that any desire [behavior] to which you are tempted at the moment is also healthy and normal. Now this, on any conceivable view, and quite apart from Christianity, must be nonsense. Surrender to all our desires obviously leads to impotence, disease, jealousies, lies, concealment, and everything that is the reverse of health, good humor, and frankness. For any happiness, even in this world, quite a lot of restraint is going to be necessary: so the claim made by every desire when it is strong, [that it is healthy and reasonable], counts for nothing. Every sane and civilized person must have some set of principles by which they choose to reject some of their desires and to permit others.

We may, indeed, be sure that perfect [behavior]—like perfect love—will not be attained by any mere human efforts. You must ask for God's help. Even when you have done so, it may seem to you for a long time that no help, or less help than you need, is being given. Never mind. After each failure, ask forgiveness, pick yourself up and try again. Very often what God first helps us towards is not the virtue itself but just this power of always trying again. For however important [your chosen behavior improvement] may be, this process [of not giving up] trains us in habits of the soul which are more

important still. It cures our illusions about ourselves and
teaches us to depend on God.

We learn, on the one hand, that we cannot trust ourselves
even in our best moments, and, on the other, that we need not
despair even in our worst, for our failures are forgiven. The
only fatal thing is to sit down content with anything less than
perfection [that is, in seeking to do what is best for us]."[15]

A favorite Jewish proverb of mine states, "Meaning is
found in limits." As I work with patients to address this
very discipline, I give them a handout with the following
homework:

> *To maintain and improve the effectiveness of my personal*
> *wellness protocol, how am I going to limit or restrain my*
> *choices and health behaviors this week? BE SPECIFIC!*
>
> *For instance, specify how you will deal with the*
> *temptations and excuses to NOT exercise, OR to just have*
> *a little taste of something NOT on the First Class or Green*
> *Light Food list.*

I also paraphrase another famous quote from C.S. Lewis as
follows:

> *Faith is the art of holding onto things your reason has once*
> *accepted in spite of your changing moods or circumstances!*
> *Take a few minutes to write out THINGS THAT YOU*
> *CAN DO that will help you to hold onto the lifestyle*
> *principles and objectives of your personal wellness protocol.*
> *FOCUS ON WHAT IS MOST IMPORTANT TO*
> *YOUR IMPROVED HEALTH.*

TO THE NURSING HOME

During the December consultation, I could sense John was a little discouraged and somewhat worn down from the entire ordeal of dealing with Mary's hospital stay and getting her moved into a rehabilitation center. But I didn't need to convince John to keep trying. Having lived more than 70 years, John was well aware of the ups and downs of life. He explained to me that this was just a temporary setback, and he was going to figure out how to get Mary back on the full protocol. We addressed the "Setting Limits" worksheet and came up with a plan.

The first challenge was how to keep Mary from being fed all the comfort foods typically served at nursing homes. She was going to be there for up to six weeks, and he didn't want Mary's symptoms of advanced Alzheimer's to return in full force. Further, if Mary's symptoms of disorientation, confusion, agitation, and hallucinations did return, John would have to move her to a more specialized rehabilitation center that was much farther away, making it hard for him to visit her twice daily.

John met with the nursing home food service director and worked out a daily meal menu for Mary. Since the best diet for brain healing avoids refined carbohydrates and meats and is loaded with dark green leafy and other colorful veggies, they tripled the normal servings of veggies and added a serving of some type of beans, peas, or lentils twice daily. They also made sure that Mary was getting a healthy amount of whole food fats (avocados, olives, nuts, seeds) on her salads or on the side.

Next on John's mind was how to get Mary exercising again. After all, Mary had a partial leg fracture and needed time to heal properly. Mary's physical therapist came to her room twice daily for rehabilitation exercises. While there,

John received permission to take Mary for slow, after-meal walks up and down the nursing home hallway.

Finally, there was the question of continuing the supplements. John had already witnessed deterioration in Mary's mental function when the recommended supplements were not taken. Knowing that nursing home administrators are concerned about medical liability issues and don't like being responsible for giving out nutritional supplements, John would need a plan.

Talking to a friend whose husband was in a memory care home, John learned that they first required a letter from their doctor outlining how each supplement was to be taken. After receiving the letter, the nurse manager explained to them that providing the nutritional supplements with each meal would require an additional charge of $650 a month!

John decided that he wouldn't fall into that trap. While visiting the nursing home to see where Mary would stay, he noticed that family members would bring in milk shakes from McDonald's or a soda and French fries from Burger King. The staff didn't have any problems with this. Since the nursing home allowed junk food to be brought in, John figured they couldn't possibly have a problem with him bringing Mary a smoothie made with organic blueberries, unsweetened almond milk, and Nanogreens (concentrated powdered green leafy veggies) blended with several tablespoons of ground up walnuts, flax seeds, and chia seeds. To bypass the medical liability concern at the nursing home, John chose to not even mention what other supplemental nutrients were also in the smoothie.

Twice daily, John brought Mary a fresh smoothie with all the brain boosting nutrients already mixed in. Several times, John noticed the staff "eyeing" the smoothie he had brought in. To this he simply smiled and said, "It's an organic blueberry and greens smoothie. I figured it would be healthier than bringing in a synthetic McDonald's milkshake that's full of high fructose corn syrup, saturated fat from unidentified sources, oxidized cholesterol, preservatives, and any number of artificial flavors."

The staff nodded slowly and agreed that John's treats for Mary were much healthier than what others were bringing to their spouses or parents.

CHAPTER 8

RISE OF THE PHOENIX

FIVE MONTHS: NEW PROGRESS

From the ashes of a failed December, John had spent the first half of January helping Mary once again become reborn. The steps taken had, for the second time, freed her from the fear and panic of Sundown Syndrome. Getting back on track had transformed Mary into a happy and functional member of her family.

Here are my notes from that phone consult:

> *Mary has been in the nursing home for 1 month. Even in this new environment she is doing much better than we anticipated. John reports that Mary will remain there for another 2 weeks. Sundowning symptoms are better. She has not talked about deceased family members while in the nursing home. Last night in passing, she talked about going upstairs to bed as she had as a child, but that was the only symptom of Sundowning. She is not experiencing*

*any anxiety, frustration or confusion. She is now
progressing in her ability to read. Today she read a more
complicated, longer word on a sign while walking in the
nursing home. During the past 3 years, she was unable to
read multi-syllable words. She is now able to tell time by
looking at the clock by her bed. In past years she was
unable to do this and wouldn't even try.*

*Mary's neurologist, noticing her dramatic improvements,
has slowly been cutting back on the Namenda. Now, at
only 5 mg, it may be stopped in next week or two. John
continues to give Mary all the proper supplements in the
smoothie. He does this twice daily when visiting Mary and
then takes her for a walk. He has only missed bringing the
smoothie 2 of the last 30 days. The nursing home is
providing a plant-based diet, but it is not fresh, only frozen
or canned. The doctor did another brain MRI on
December 18, and he reports that the scan suggests that
there is no way she should be able to function cognitively.
He is amazed at her improvements.*

Six Months: Goodbye Sundown, Hello Sunrise

Mary was eventually able to return home from the nursing
home, and her condition continued to improve. If there
ever was a fitting euphemism for Alzheimer's, it is
Sundown Syndrome. It goes far beyond the fearful
symptoms that often occur an hour or more before
sundown until bedtime. It also relates to a time of life
where physical and emotional health is rapidly dimming as
if the sun is going down on the very ability to function as
normal human beings. Even the most basic daily activities
that we all take for granted are at risk of being

compromised. After the consultation, I also recorded the following clinical notes:

Since being in the rehabilitation nursing home for over a month, Mary sometimes expresses concern about being left alone at times, but mostly because John had to leave her for parts of the day and when going back home to sleep. We reviewed multiple labs. The neurologist started Mary on low-dose Levothyroxine in early October, and Mary has taken this for just over 4 months. Thyroid is much better with TSH improving from 3.91 to 1.81. However, her main thyroid hormone, the Free T3, is still low normal at 2.3 from 2.1. This still represents an area that needs to improve in order to further optimize brain health. The goal is for Free T3 to get it into the upper half of normal (>3.1). We also want the Free T4 in the upper half of normal, but its currently still in the lower third of normal. John has agreed to share the new labs with Mary's neurologist and request an increase in the prescription dose of Levothyxoxine. We can retest again in 2 months. This is to further optimize cognition and cardiovascular health.

No Sundown Syndrome present anymore. Avoiding the "white foods" and refined products as per the protocol greatly helped along with the supplements to initially address the sundowning. While in the nursing home, the supplements were not given about 25% of the time, and this did impact cognition adversely as she was less responsive cognitively.

Currently, for exercise, the physical therapist comes twice weekly. John had sciatic pain until yesterday, so the walking sessions have been on hold till today. The goal is to get back to 5 days per week walking at the grocery store for 30+ minutes, as before. They walk together in the produce section and almond milk sections but wisely avoid the sugary areas. It was very helpful to use pineapple to mask the taste of the powders from the 12 opened capsules in each smoothie. John continues to use a colorful cup, lid, and straw, so that she can't see the contents. Doing smoothies 3 times daily allows Mary to get all supplements down easily.

Communication is now more fluent with more complete sentences compared to when she was initially improving and able to only say a few words followed by jibber jabber. John is now able to clearly understand everything Mary is saying. Prior to the protocol there was no communication. After 3 months, words started to come out. About 1 month ago, [Mary] started communicating thoughts with clear sentences. Mary is able to read headlines of paper or magazines when John is reading them sitting near her. She is able to recognize the hour on the wall clock but does not recognize the minutes yet. Mary is now showing emotion by smiling and laughing with others and even progressing further since the last consult. Clothes are fitting better. No signs of anxiety or frustration are present now.

Nothing can bring more joy to a spouse than to see their life partner of four to five decades, whose very light of life has been fading for years, be transformed into a sentient human being again. With a twinkle in their eye, John and Mary were now able to converse and share heartfelt recognition of their times together; both past and present.

The sun seemed to be setting for an eternal night but now it had risen, showcasing a new day with renewed possibilities. There was still a large measure of cognitive decline, but it had improved more than either of them had dared to hope. Gradually but steadily, cognitive decline had reversed. They were now able to look into each other's eyes, experiencing a revived relationship and feeling of rekindled love. The sunrise of hope had brought joy, warmth, and other familiar emotions back into their lives.

SUCCESSFUL HALT OF NAMENDA

Towards the end of the hour-long phone consultation, John paused a moment to reflect on Mary's metamorphosis in just a little more than six months.

"In my enthusiasm to report all of Mary's improvements," John explained, "I totally forgot to tell you. Just last week, Mary's neurologist completely stopped Mary's only remaining Alzheimer's medication."

Mary was now off the Namenda (also referred to by its generic name Memantine). Mary had been on that medication for more than three years without any sign of benefit with the doctor noting a continued decline in cognitive function while on the highest dose. The doctor acknowledged that clearly the comprehensive and personalized risk-management strategies used during the previous six months were responsible for Mary's dramatic cognitive improvements.

The doctor had put his hand on John's shoulder, looked into his eyes, and said, *"You* did this, John. It's because of your commitment to Mary that she is so much better. Mary could not have done this without you."

Pausing a moment, the doctor had smiled and then chuckled, saying, "There is nothing in the conventional medical literature even remotely suggesting this is possible. Certainly not when factoring in how severe Mary's symptoms were. Whatever you have been doing, don't stop, for this has defied expectation at every turn."

DEFYING THE VERDICT

Norman Cousins, in his book *Anatomy of an Illness,* wrote, "Don't deny the diagnosis, defy the verdict." John had fully embraced Mary's diagnosis of Alzheimer's, but he hadn't accepted the verdict. He had defied the notion that there was nothing he could do. He had found a guide—a light shining on the dark path to help him navigate the journey from sundown to sunrise.

TURNING BACK TIME

Walking out of the neurology clinic that day with Mary holding onto his arm, John started to smile. He was thinking about how he'd felt walking out of the same office six months earlier.

The casual onlookers who were sitting in the waiting room saw John wiping tears from his face, but then they noticed his big smile. His tears came from a cathartic release culminating from all his hopes and dreams for Mary. What he had done to stop Mary's sun from going down completely had been worth every effort. John could hardly believe it. They had actually turned back time— more than five years-worth of time, to be exact.

John realized that if he could just hold onto Mary's current improvements, he would be very happy. But somehow he knew that more blessings were on the way. Seeing Mary improve had changed him too. Joy had replaced despair in his heart, giving him a renewed emotional energy. It was as if he was getting a foretaste—a sliver of fruit—from the tree of life!

Driving home that afternoon, his smile broadened as he mouthed the words of a now favorite proverb, "Hope deferred maketh the heart sick; but when the desire cometh, it is a tree of life."[16]

COST OF ALZHEIMER'S

Later in our phone call, I offered to review all of Mary's supplemental herbs and nutrients and prioritize them in case they were getting tired of taking so many supplements. John quickly countered that using the smoothie to combine all the supplements three times a day was simple enough and much less of a hassle or burden compared to the three to four hours of agitation and life disruption associated with her past symptoms of Sundown Syndrome.

When I asked John whether he had concerns about the monthly cost and wanted to further prioritize the supplements in order to lower the expense, he declined. He didn't want to minimize or lose the improvements Mary had achieved so far. John mentioned that when looking into the expense of placing Mary into a residential memory care facility, he learned it would cost him more than $100,000 a year.

John knew that, as Alzheimer's progresses, the average patient with advanced Alzheimer's requires three different people to provide care covering three eight-hour shifts. The intensive care required is time-consuming and is a tremendous emotional and economic burden on spouse, family, and society. John had recognized seven months earlier that Mary had reached the advanced stage of Alzheimer's. The challenge was that he was the only one taking care of her, which greatly limited his sleep and personal time.

"The cost of following Mary's personalized wellness protocol is just a fraction of the what it would cost me if we weren't on the protocol," John said.

Regardless, I encouraged John to make a full list of supplements and ingredients, including pictures of the front and back of the bottles, so that we could fully review them at the next visit and see whether there were any excess or overlap that needed to be adjusted. It is important to fully justify each supplement based on the current nutritional science and peer-reviewed literature and that they be appropriate based on past lab findings, medical risk factors, and medical history.

EIGHT MONTHS: MORE PROGRESS

After eight months, I recorded the following clinical notes concerning Mary's progress and further reviewed her supplement list.

> *Mary ran out of Levothyroxin 25 mcg last Friday, so she has been off her thyroid medication for 5 days. I strongly recommended staying on the neurologist's Rx as per last month's notes and encouraged him to increase the dose as we discussed previously. In future we may need to work with her doctor to add very low dose Cytomel in order optimize the Free T3 thyroid hormone. Fully reviewed supplement list. Based on the degree of cognitive improvement we adjusted doses including cutting back on the therapeutic herbs Gotu Kola, Ashwaganda and Bacopa to only once daily.*

NINE MONTHS: A BAD FALL

At nine months into the protocol, Mary had to go to the emergency room after falling out of bed at 2 o'clock in the morning. She had no broken bones but did have lower back pain. The physician on duty said she was badly bruised but saw no sign of lasting damage other than pain. I recorded the following in my clinical notes:

> *Mary trembles when walking now but today was able to walk to the dinner table without support. She never likes to just sit but likes to walk from one end of the ranch style house to the other end. Mary does this back and forth 4 times lasting 30 minutes and repeats this 3 times daily. The ER doctor took multiple X-rays of legs and back because of constant leg and lower back pain. He found no sign of skeletal problem that would limit her ability to walk.*

SIDE EFFECTS OF PAIN MEDICATION

As a matter of hospital protocol, Mary was offered the opioid Oxycodone for pain management, but John refused. John was well aware of the potential decline in cognitive ability associated with using opioid pain medications.[17] He chose instead to focus on optimizing natural anti-inflammatory supplements. The last thing John needed was to see Mary's improvements in brain function fade away because of poor choices in medication management.

ANTI-INFLAMMATORY BENEFITS OF CURCUMIN, DHA, AND CBD

I discussed with John natural strategies for lowering Mary's inflammation, and we discussed pain management. We added pharmaceutical grade, 95 percent standardized curcumin at two 400 mg capsules three times daily to Mary's mealtime smoothies. We also temporarily doubled Mary's normal dose of DHA/EPA Omega 3 oils. Finally, we added a high-quality, nano-emulsified form of CBD oil—one of the most powerful nutritional supports for inflammation, pain, and anxiety. CBD is the active ingredient of hemp oil.[18] CBD Cannabinoids are non-psychogenic, yet contain highly therapeutic compounds derived from hemp oil that have documented neuroprotective and anti-inflammatory benefits. CBD also powerfully limits damage to brain cells caused by beta amyloid plaque.[19]

DOCTOR AMAZED AT IMPROVEMENT

John shared with me that Mary's doctor continued to be amazed at her improvement over time. Her neurologist retested her cognition. I recorded the following in my clinical notes:

> *Mary's improvements have been stable since last month. No Sundown Syndrome recurrence. At times, there is some passing mention about possible visits from relatives that have already passed on. Time awareness when looking at the clock now includes correct assessment of the minute on a digital clock. With an analog clock she can tell hour but not minutes at this time. This continued to improve this month. Mary's ability to communicate is also getting better. She is able to point to things and describe them. At times she is able to talk back and forth with John with good, complete and understandable sentences. Mary had not been able to do this for 3 years. She is also now able to communicate with others at home. This includes talking 10-15 minutes on the phone when her sister calls. At church Mary is now able to respond to those who speak to her. In the past Mary just acted as if she didn't hear them. They saw the neurologist this week. The MoCA cognition*

test is still at 0/30; but the doctor marvels at her improvements, "Based on the literature, there is no way Mary's daily functional abilities should have improved so dramatically." John is starting to work with Mary on a daily basis to draw a clock and practice brain testing. Their doctor also approved increasing the Levothyroid hormone to 50 mcg daily and will see them again in three months.

As I hung up the phone that day, roughly nine months since John and I had first talked, I too had a smile on my face. Few things are more satisfying to any doctor than seeing someone overcome seemingly overwhelming odds.

CHAPTER 9

LIFE TO YEARS OR YEARS TO LIFE?

In 2017, I was privileged to present this information to the annual conference of the American College of Lifestyle Medicine (ACLM). Because of the great interest in this topic, I was asked to write a paper for the *American Journal of Lifestyle Medicine.* With the help of Paulina Shetty, a nutritionist and director of education for ACLM, our paper, "Clinical Lifestyle Medicine Strategies for Preventing and Reversing Memory Loss in Alzheimer's," was published in May of 2018.[20] I have included a portion of that paper in this book.

Patients often express to clinicians that they do not want to live long lives because they assume that it will extend the years of dysfunction associated with chronic diseases and, in particular, Alzheimer's Disease. This, of course, is generally true for those who do not believe in the power of lifestyle medicine to prevent, treat, and even reverse disease. Fortunately, lifestyle medicine is uniquely suited to guide the aging population of patients who are open to evaluating and broadly addressing the underlying risk factors associated with Alzheimer's.

SENIOR MOMENTS

Many individuals are under the impression that experiencing "senior moments" and serious mental decline are just a normal part of aging and that there is nothing that can be done to prevent, let alone treat or reverse, cognitive decline. With no current hope for prevention or successful care, those experiencing mental decline tend to delay or even avoid seeking medical attention altogether. Patients who do seek medical care may also avoid disclosing their symptoms to their doctors out of fear of losing their work clearance, drivers' license, or independence altogether.

MARGINAL, UNSUSTAINED, SYMPTOMATIC EFFECT

Why should anyone think differently? So far, standard medical care has proven to be rather unsuccessful in the treatment of Alzheimer's, and part of that failure may be attributed to the methods. Currently, conventional medicine treats Alzheimer's with a one-step approach, which typically consists of prescribing cognition-enhancing medication such as Namenda. Unfortunately, the current approach to treating Alzheimer's provides nothing more than a marginal, unsustained, symptomatic effect, with little or no effect on disease progression itself. The main fallacy of this approach in treating Alzheimer's is that it does not treat the cause of disease, nor does it begin to address the multiple risk factors of Alzheimer's.

THUMB TACK RULES

The conventional methods of addressing Alzheimer's can be compared to the following "thumb tack rules," as postulated by Dr. Sid Baker, Professor Emeritus, Yale University School of Medicine. "If you are sitting on a tack, it takes a lot of aspirin to make it feel good.[21] If you are sitting on two tacks, removing just one does not result in a 50 percent improvement." [22]

But what if someone is sitting on 36 tacks? Addressing and removing only five tacks is not going to make the person feel better or provide much improvement at all. The same goes with the standard medical approach to Alzheimer's. If we only address one risk factor at a time, there will be minimal benefit. But by comprehensively addressing and treating all known risk factors for Alzheimer's, clinical experience and research shows that signs and symptoms of mild cognitive impairment and early Alzheimer's can often be reversed.[23]

The field of lifestyle medicine is unique in its ability to meet the demands of the above injunction. What if, instead of experiencing fear of a diagnosis or of losing independence, people could experience hope?

Remember, "Don't deny the diagnosis, defy the verdict."[24] The goal is to embrace the diagnosis and then develop an aggressive intervention plan.

DETERMINING RISK FACTORS

To attain effective improvements in Alzheimer's, one must identify risk factors, address the underlying causes, and focus on a combination of functional and lifestyle medicine strategies that provide a comprehensive, programmatic, and network-based approach that is sufficient to achieve epigenetic transformation and neurologic healing through multiple and necessary synergistic components. To promote optimal health and enable healing, research neurologist Dr. Dale Bredesen has developed a clinical protocol that focuses on a multifaceted approach to treating Alzheimer's. This protocol aims to provide all the necessary elements that optimize cognition while also removing any of the elements that interfere with cognition.

CHAPTER 10

TENETS OF THE BREDESEN PROTOCOL

STUDIES PUBLISHED BY DR. DALE BREDESEN and the UCLA Center for Alzheimer's Research have documented that mild cognitive impairment and early Alzheimer's may often be reversed within six months after initiating a comprehensive, functional, and lifestyle medicine–focused program.[25] The basic tenets and themes of the comprehensive therapeutic system often referred to as the Bredesen Protocol include the following:

1. In Alzheimer's treatment, there is not a single drug that gives anything beyond a marginal, unsustained, symptomatic effect, with little or no effect on disease progression.
2. In order to get effective improvements in Alzheimer's, we must address the many underlying causes of the disease and focus on a combination of therapeutic strategies. This is a comprehensive, network-based, synergistic approach.

3. It will be necessary to target multiple pathways simultaneously in order to stimulate improvement in symptoms and pathophysiology.

4. The goal is not simply to normalize metabolic parameters such as lab values and other risk factors, but rather to optimize them. It is important to understand that laboratory reference ranges typically include values found in 95% of the general public. Having lab values within the reference range, therefore, is not a sensitive or effective standard for health risk assessment. An optimal lab value would be associated with the healthiest individuals within the population and represent those who are least likely to develop Alzheimer's over time. (For a thorough explanation on normal vs optimal lab values, read Chapter 12 "Testing...Testing.. Choosing the Best Clinical Lab Tests" in my book, *Hello Healthy*.)

5. Just as in other chronic diseases, the goal is to reach a threshold effect—a tipping point—such that, once enough of the underlying causal network of risk factors have been optimized, the pathological process would be halted or even reversed.

6. The approach is personalized based on more than 100 data points, including lab testing, MRI brain scans, genomic evaluation, cognitive testing that includes the Montreal Cognitive Assessment, and a detailed medical and family history.

7. Each network risk factor is addressed in the most rational physiological way and as far upstream

in the cause-effect chain as possible. Lifestyle medicine and clinical nutrition strategies are the core interventional approaches to therapy.

8. The protocol has continued optimization over time. Previous lab tests that were not optimal should be retested at appropriate intervals, initially after 2 to 3 months to see whether the current interventions are adequate. If not, changes are made and the labs in question are repeated again in 2 to 3 months. This is repeated until optimization or an acceptable improvement has occurred. Thereafter, labs may be repeated every 6 to 12 months as needed.

GENETIC TESTING AND THE PERSONALIZED GENOMIC PROFILE

The first and most important component of the Bredesen Protocol is to complete comprehensive laboratory testing and a genomic profile. One of the easiest and most affordable ways to test for Alzheimer's-related gene mutations is to order a Health and Ancestry gene saliva test at *www.23andme.com*. The genomic profile and lab testing assist in revealing the underlying and specific risk factors that over time promote cognitive decline and Alzheimer's. The Bredesen Protocol encourages a broad evaluation of genetic mutations but specifically analyzes the following genes: ApoE, MTHFR, APP, BDNF, PSEN1, and PSEN2. I encourage a more comprehensive genetic review that includes providing each patient with a 20+ page personalized genomic report.

Each of us has many genetic mutations that can be discovered by this type of genetic testing. Knowing which of your genes carry significant mutations helps your doctor or specialist determine which biochemical pathways in your body and brain are compromised. Genetic mutations cause errors in the formation of enzymes, which make these enzymes misshapen and therefore less functional and much less effective in properly activating their specific metabolic and biochemical pathways.

As one example, many people have a defective Glutamate Decarboxylase (GAD) gene. The GAD gene mutation codes for the production of a GAD enzyme that is misshapen and therefore much less functional in its ability to properly break down glutamate into GABA. In my practice, I recommend genomic testing to every patient and frequently see double copy mutations of GAD. This mutation limits the conversion of glutamate, which is the dominant excitatory neurotransmitter in the brain, into the most calming neurotransmitter in the brain called GABA.

When we experience a high level of stress or anxiety, an excessive amount of the excitatory neurotransmitter glutamate builds up in the nervous system. If allowed to stay high, glutamate will have neurotoxic effects on the brain. This glutamate storm can cause significant damage and even death of brain cells.[26] Chronic stress, when not managed effectively, will lead to chronic glutamate toxicity, triggering neurodegenerative diseases and in particular damage to the memory centers promoting Alzheimer's.[27]

But God has created the body in a special way. The GAD enzyme present in our nerves can effectively turn Glutamate into GABA. Yes, that's right. This little miracle enzyme can take a neurotoxic level of glutamate and instantly transform it into the calming and protective neurotransmitter GABA. However, like most miracles, there are conditions that must be met. In this case, there must be an adequate level of vitamin B6 for the conversion to occur. When the GAD enzyme is misshapen because of a GAD mutation, it will require much more vitamin B6 to catalyze the enzymatic reaction and effectively convert glutamate to GABA. It is all basic biochemistry. This is a key example of why some people require substantially more of a particular vitamin or mineral than indicated by the Recommended Dietary Allowances (RDA's).

Genetic Mutations & Brain Shrinkage

Mutations in the MTHFR, FOLR, MTRR, or BHMT genes can individually or collectively decrease the ability of the enzymes that the genes code for to break down and metabolize homocysteine. This is a major reason for elevated blood levels of homocysteine, which is neurotoxic above optimal levels. Comparing elderly who have normal cognition with elderly who have Mild Cognitive Impairment or Alzheimer's, researchers discovered that elevated homocysteine levels were strongly related to smaller hippocampal volume. This is the area of the brain controlling the conversion of short-term memory into long-term memory.[28] Cognitive decline occurs when a large number of hippocampal brain cells die and are not replaced by new brain cells. This causes the hippocampus to shrink over time and is referred to as hippocampal volume loss.

Large studies show that even mild elevation of blood homocysteine increases risk of neurodegenerative diseases such as mild cognitive impairment, Alzheimer's, vascular dementia, and even stroke. As homocysteine levels rise, the risk of brain toxicity and damage increases in a dose-dependent manner. Recent studies in which elderly were supplemented with B vitamins "demonstrated a slowing of brain atrophy and improvement in some domains of cognitive function."[29]

A 2017 case-control study showed that individuals with folate vitamin levels in the lower third of the population were three times more likely to have Mild Cognitive Impairment (MCI) and almost three-and-a-half times more likely to have Alzheimer's than those who had folate levels in the upper third of the population. Conversely, those with homocysteine blood levels in the upper third of the population average were almost 3 times more likely to have MCI and 3.6 times more likely to have Alzheimer's compared with those who had homocysteine levels in the lowest third of the population average.[30]

"A 5-year study of people older than 60 years showed that percentage brain volume loss occurred at an average rate of 0.7% ± 0.3% per year. However, the decrease in brain volume was greater among those with lower vitamin B12 levels. For those with the lowest tertile of baseline vitamin B12 (<308 pmol/L [or < 417 pg/mL for lab tests done in the US]), there was a six-fold increase in the rate of brain volume loss."[31] Older adults who live independently in their community also have smaller brain hippocampuses if their homocysteine levels are elevated.[32][33]

At this point, I must emphasize the importance of testing levels of these vitamins in your blood. I frequently see patients who think they are doing everything right, but they actually have up to a 600 percent greater risk of brain shrinkage and resulting dementia simply because they are unaware of their risk due to a "normal" but lower than optimal level of vitamin B12. I encourage my patients to consistently maintain B12 levels in the upper third of normal. At least >700 and preferably >900 pg/mL. I also encourage patients to get their blood homocysteine levels into the 6 to 8 umol/L range. Not everyone can get their levels down into this optimal range, but every point improvement helps lower the risk.

Lowering homocysteine blood levels using vitamins B12, B6, and folate is a reasonable step in decreasing neurotoxicity, thus improving the potential for other strategies to heal damaged neurons and even replace dead neurons with newly-formed brain cells.

COMPREHENSIVE LABORATORY TESTING

A patient's tendency to follow a destructive inflammatory pattern compared with a healing neurologically protective pattern is assessed by labs including the following: high-sensitivity CRP; interleukin-6; tumor necrosis factor–α; homocysteine; vitamin B6; vitamin B12; folate; vitamin D as 25-OH-D; vitamin C; vitamin E; omega 6:3 ratio; a comprehensive metabolic panel that includes albumin, globulin, creatinine, blood urea nitrogen, estimated glomerular filtration rate, glucose, calcium, and potassium; NMR LipoProfile that includes the low-density lipoprotein (LDL) cholesterol particle number; small LDL particle number; and LDL size as well as all the components of the standard lipid profile that include total, LDL, and high-density lipoprotein cholesterol and triglycerides; total glutathione; and hemoglobin A1c.

Additionally, because insulin resistance is one of the most significant metabolic drivers toward cognitive decline and Alzheimer's, I recommend a 4-hour Glucose Tolerance tTest, which also assesses blood levels of insulin at fasting, 1 hour, and 2 hours and assesses cortisol levels at fasting, 3 hours, and 4 hours.

Trophic factors are hormones that promote growth and healing balance. Assessment of trophic factors includes testing estradiol, progesterone, pregnenolone, cortisol,

DHEA-sulfate, testosterone, free testosterone, and a comprehensive thyroid profile, including thyroid stimulating hormone, free T4, free T3, reverse T3, thyroid peroxidase antibody, and thyroglobulin antibody. The goal is to promote strategies that optimize each hormone tested.

Additionally, screening for exposure to toxic metals or imbalances of nutrient elements in whole blood is recommended. The elements evaluated with this test are calcium, copper, lithium, magnesium, manganese, molybdenum, selenium, and zinc as well as potentially toxic elements such as arsenic, cadmium, cobalt, lead, mercury, silver, and strontium. Finally, additional lab tests for mold and other biotoxin-related causes of cognitive impairment are also assessed in the Bredesen Protocol.

Once comprehensive genetic and laboratory tests are completed, the Bredesen Protocol promotes a diet composed primarily of whole plant foods. It optimizes sleep patterns, personalizes an exercise program, and addresses other factors that, when combined together into a comprehensive therapeutic program, have collectively produced subjective and objective cognitive improvements in the vast majority of participants.

THE SIX SUBTYPES OF ALZHEIMER'S

With more than 150 data points generated by the above screening process, it is possible to complete metabolic profiling and to determine how significantly each of the six subtypes of Alzheimer's is contributing to cognitive decline. By establishing which subtypes are predominant, it is possible to tailor the protocol for each patient. Dr. Bredesen summarizes the subtypes below:[34] [35]

TYPE 1, INFLAMMATORY. This type is associated with inflammatory markers such as high-sensitivity CRP. The inflammation may be a result of infections, suboptimal diet, or other factors. Risk for type 1 is increased by ApoE4, chronic infections, transfats, and other factors.

Type 1.5, GLYCOTOXIC. Type 1.5 has features of both type 1 (inflammatory) and type 2 (atrophic). In this type, chronically high glucose levels damage multiple proteins, cells, and tissues, leading to inflammation and auto-antibodies, all of which increase the risk for type 1 Alzheimer's. Meanwhile, the responding high insulin levels and associated insulin resistance reduce the trophic effects of insulin and increase risk for type 2. Risk for type 1.5 is increased by ApoE4, type 2 diabetes, and prediabetes.

TYPE 2, ATROPHIC. This type is associated with especially rapid reduction in trophic support such as estradiol, testosterone, insulin, vitamin D, and neurotrophins. Risk for type 2 is increased by ApoE4, early hysterectomy/oophorectomy without hormone replacement, low vitamin D levels, and in some cases menopause/andropause. It is important to rule out sleep apnea as well.

TYPE 3, TOXIC. Type 3 is quite different from types 1, 1.5, and 2 and often presents with features other than (or in addition to) memory loss, such as depression and problems in calculating, organizing, following instructions, or word finding. Type 3 is associated with exposure to toxins (dementogens) such as mercury, high copper levels, anesthetics, mycotoxins (toxins produced by molds), or tick-related toxins (e.g., from Lyme disease). Risk for type 3 is not increased and may even be decreased by ApoE4.

TYPE 4, VASCULAR. We used to think of vascular disease as being unrelated to Alzheimer's, but over the past several years it has become clear that vascular abnormalities contribute importantly to Alzheimer's. In type 4, chronic vascular disease may be associated with high homocysteine, vascular amyloid, or breach of the blood-brain barrier (among other contributors), and all are associated with the development of Alzheimer's.

Type 5, TRAUMATIC. When the brain is traumatized, for example, as a result of an auto accident, the amyloid associated with Alzheimer's is produced as a response. Trauma is thus a risk factor for Alzheimer's. In many cases, the amyloid is removed, followed by chronic traumatic encephalopathy. We now know that chronic traumatic encephalopathy is common in football players and in other contact sports, as was featured in the film "Concussion." Type 5 typically lacks amyloid but is related to Alzheimer's in featuring neurofibrillary tangles made of the τ-protein.

CHAPTER 11

PATIENT ZERO: BREDESEN CASE STUDY

In Bredesen's groundbreaking 2014 paper, he presented 10 case studies of patients with cognitive decline. Three were diagnosed with Subjective Cognitive Decline. These individuals could score normally on a cognitive/memory assessment but reported that their mental capacity had declined over the last few years. Four of the ten were diagnosed with Mild Cognitive Impairment, and five had early to late forms of Alzheimer's Disease. All but the one patient who had advanced Alzheimer's showed clear improvement in cognitive function after following the comprehensive program for 6 to 12 months. This demonstrated that a process of ongoing reversal of cognitive decline had been activated and maintained during the study.

This next case study is drawn from Dr. Bredesen's research. To obtain and read the information firsthand, search the Internet for "UCLA Alzheimer's Study." The entire study in PDF format may be downloaded by searching for "Reversal of Cognitive Decline: a novel therapeutic program" published September 2014 in the journal *Aging*.[36] It contains a great deal of information, much of which is not in lay terms; however, focusing on the actual recommendations in the case study can be very helpful.

This patient is also referred to as "Patient Zero" because it was her devastating initial cognitive decline and then her dramatic reversal back to her previous functional professional capacity that officially started the clinical application of lifestyle and functional medicine strategies now referred to as "The Bredesen Protocol." This protocol now gives hope where previously there was only a diagnosis of despair.

Patient Zero was a 67-year-old traveling business analyst, a brilliant lady (BL) who in the last two years had experienced significant and progressive memory loss. She was no longer able to analyze complex data and prepare complex reports for corporate leaders. BL was traveling all over the country engaging in these tasks when all of a sudden she realized she was no longer able to complete the multifaceted cognitive job requirements.

Previously, BL could type up detailed reports on the fly, emailing the documents to the board of directors and fully satisfying her contractual obligations. However, cognitive decline had progressed so swiftly that BL could no longer even remember four-digit number codes, a skill she had possessed before. When back at home for a few nights, she would sit down to read something interesting. Often when she reached the bottom of the page, BL realized she had no idea what she had just read.

BL was having increasing problems remembering recent things she had done. Just navigating around the neighborhood, she'd be driving along looking at the streets and then totally miss the street she was supposed to turn on. BL may have turned at the same corner for the past 10 years, yet now she missed the turn.

BL's memory was becoming a serious problem. She started calling her pets by wrong names. Even when she was getting up in the night to use the restroom, BL would feel for the light switch only to realize there was no light switch where she expected it to be. These memory losses started worrying her, so BL went to her doctor.

After BL explained what was going on, her doctor actually said to her, "Well, you know your mother had memory problems when she was in her early 60s." This was BL's greatest fear; she had seen her mother gradually progress into severe dementia. BL's mother had lived in a nursing home for almost 20 years because of dementia before passing away in her early 80s.

BL did not want to live the life her mother had experienced. She had personally witnessed her mom's decline for 20 years. BL was fearful of receiving the dreaded diagnosis but still poured out her heart to the doctor. Her doctor told her, "Well, you know your mother had this problem; you have all the symptoms. There's nothing we can do for you." BL left the medical office that day feeling very discouraged.

HOPE FOR REVERSAL

When it came to medication management, BL's doctor was 100 percent correct; there was essentially nothing valid or worth doing according to the pharmaceutical research. BL was so upset that she immediately tried to obtain long-term care insurance, but of course the insurance company did their homework. That is their job. They pulled the charts from all BL's medical visits and saw BL's doctor had recorded "memory problems" in her chart. BL's application for long-term care insurance was "denied."

Facing a future without the cognitive ability to stay employed and without long-term care insurance like her mother had had, BL knew she could no longer survive financially and ultimately felt suicide was her best option. Thankfully, before acting on her decision, she reached out to her best high school friend to commiserate. She basically said, "You know, this is my last hoorah. I can't live like this. I can't live expecting what I know is about to happen." Very concerned for BL's happiness, her friend made her an appointment to see Dr. Bredesen.

Even though BL felt she did not have any hope, she went to the appointment because her friend had encouraged her to go. BL learned from Bredesen's personalized wellness protocol about strategies she could follow that would lower her specific risk factors for Alzheimer's. For the first time, BL started to believe that there was hope. BL gladly followed her new protocol.

Over time, to BL's amazement all her symptoms of cognitive decline abated; she was now able to prepare reports again and navigate without problems. She could read and retain information and even remember phone numbers. Overall, she had become asymptomatic! She was now functional again and was able to continue to work, thus maintaining a high level of financial independence.

BL noted that her memory was better now than it had been in many years! Sometime later, BL contracted an acute viral illness—a bad cold. Feeling terribly ill, BL decided to discontinue her personalized wellness protocol until she was better. Unfortunately, and very quickly, she began experiencing a decline of her mental capacity. Dementia was coming back!

BL realized she had to get back to the wellness protocol that had previously helped her. As soon as BL reinstated the strategies, the dementia she was re-experiencing completely reversed itself. Five years later at age 73, BL continues working full-time and remains completely asymptomatic. So, what are the questions you should be asking? What did she do? Could this apply to me also? What can I do to personalize the Bredesen Protocol for myself?

Personalized Wellness Strategies

BL's therapeutic wellness program, taken straight from her journal, included the *elimination of all simple carbohydrates*. For some people this may seem to be fanatical; however, this is one of the most critical steps in preventing further cognitive decline and in supporting the brain's natural healing potential. Anyone who is not willing to optimize their diet and make multiple changes in their lifestyle will not be able to accomplish the positive results they hope for.

In addition to cutting out all simple carbohydrates, BL *eliminated all processed foods*. Foods can be divided into first class, second class, and third class. More information about food classes is available in my book *Goodbye Diabetes*.[i]

Thirdly, BL decided to *eliminate gluten* in her program. Not everyone on the program needs to eliminate gluten; the protocol should be personalized and adapted to individual needs. BL also dramatically *increased her vegetable and fruit intake,* and fifthly, started a *stress reduction program*. She began paying attention to her lifestyle choices and implementing a conscious plan to manage stress by

---

[i] See *Goodbye Diabetes*, chapter 13 "Be a First-Class Foodie", pp. 144-161, author Dr. Wes Youngberg. Available winwellness.org.

focusing on the good things in life. Stopping to "smell the roses" and carve out a section of each day to do something special for yourself and those you love is an effective strategy in helping to reduce stress.

A sixth decision BL made was to not just work, work, work. She *increased her sleep time* from a typical 4 to 5 hour night to 7 to 8 hours of sleep per night.[ii]

IMPORTANCE OF SLEEP IN DEMENTIA REVERSAL

Nearly everyone who has participated in this life-changing program and experienced successful reversal of cognitive symptoms has by necessity developed and implemented a plan to get adequate sleep. Most who struggle with sleep problems find it difficult to figure out the underlying factors involved. Your brain cannot detoxify if you do not sleep well. And if you cannot detoxify the brain, you are not going to get rid of the toxic beta amyloid plaque buildup.

Researchers are now telling us that, based on available scans and multiple studies, by the time we are age 40 most of us already have visible, measurable levels of beta amyloid plaque in our brains.

Yes, it is true. When you sleep, you can get rid of beta amyloid plaque. Detoxification of the brain occurs when you sleep soundly, when you sleep deeply, and when you sleep properly. Adequate quality sleep is critically important to the healing of the brain.

BL took melatonin, half a milligram at bedtime, to actually increase deep sleep. Not everyone needs melatonin, and not everyone can handle taking melatonin without unwanted side effects. Remember, each program is

---

[ii] See Dr. Wes Youngberg's book *Hello Healthy,* Chapter 11, "Rest Is Best", pp. 221-239. Available winwellness.org or dryoungberg.com.

individualized, and the decision to use melatonin should be determined after discussing the pros and cons with your doctor. Melatonin can be a common-sense supplement to try, especially if sleep is a problem.

VITAMIN SUPPLEMENTS AND BRAIN HEALTH

The seventh strategy BL chose for her wellness protocol was to take 1,000 micrograms daily of methylcobalamin, which is a special form of vitamin B12. Taking a B12 supplement is a prudent recommendation for anyone who is vegetarian, especially if their diet is 100 percent plant-based. However, it really does not matter how much dairy or animal products you consume. Chances are that you also need more vitamin B12 in the form of a supplement.

Unfortunately, an erroneous idea exists about the vegan and plant-based community regarding the need for supplemental B12. The suggestion is that if you need a supplement, it's because your diet isn't healthy. This is in my opinion an absolute misapplication of the science. In other words, vegan or non-vegan, everyone should be getting some supplemental B12.

Years ago, a large multi-university research study yielded results indicating that if you had a Vitamin B12 level in the normal range, but it was in the lower third of the normal range, your risk of Alzheimer's and a senile brain increased. Autopsies literally demonstrated a 600 percent increased likelihood of a shrunken brain.[37] This is the very definition of senility. Senility simply means that the brain has lost so many neurons and synapses that it has literally shrunk enough to be clearly noticeable on brain MRI scans.

The same principle applies to the eighth strategy BL chose for her wellness protocol—vitamin D supplements.

BL took vitamin D3 at 2,000 International Units daily. In my opinion, this is an inadequate dose; however, as BL personalized her own protocol, she, as her own 'chairperson of the board,' chose to take 2,000 IUs, which is more than twice the officially recommended dose.[iii]

BL also took 2,000 milligrams of fish oil daily. An equivalent to fish oil is now available as a pure, toxin free, vegan product in a marine algae-based supplement. One of the keys for brain health is to consume at least 1,000 milligrams of DHA daily. In addition, you may also take up to 1,000 mg of EPA. Don't confuse this with the total amount of oil in the capsules, since two thirds of the oil is typically NOT from the therapeutic DHA or EPA fatty acids.

A supplement such as this is recommended for anyone, including vegans or people who are 100 percent plant-based. Keep in mind that you will not get DHA or EPA in any substantial or clinically relevant quantity by converting chia seeds, walnuts, or any other form of omega-3 into the specifically beneficial forms of DHA and EPA. I am not downplaying the benefits or importance of chia seeds, flax seeds, or walnuts in any way. These foods are very valuable to your health, but although they do contain healthy Omega-3 fats, they will not generate sufficient DHA or EPA necessary to protect the brain against oxidative and inflammatory stresses that are driving Alzheimer's risk in most of us.

BL's doctor also recommended she take CoQ10, 200 milligrams daily. CoQ10 is a supplement that provides protection to our brain and heart by optimizing the function of mitochondria within every cell. Mitochondria

---

[iii] For a more complete discussion of vitamin D, see WIN! Wellness, Book 1, *Getting Started*, Chapter 4, "The Miracle Drug—Sunlight" pp. 50-64, coauthor Dr. Wes Youngberg. Available winwellness.org and dryoungberg.com.

are the small structures within all cells that act as energy generators by converting fats and carbohydrates into ATP – the currency of energy within our body.

BL's ninth strategy for her wellness protocol was to exercise for 30 minutes or more four to six times per week. Exercise can improve all aspects of health. Many studies are now suggesting that exercise should be at the top of the list of the fundamental strategies to improve brain health. No matter our physical condition, each one of us can work with our health care team to develop an exercise program that is uniquely appropriate for us. Exercise also helps us feel better right away and therefore makes it much more likely that we will also address the other areas of our personalized wellness protocol, including optimizing diet, sleep, stress, and the other beneficial strategies.

CONNECTION BETWEEN SENILITY AND EXERCISE

Senility refers to shrinkage of an organ or tissue in question. Why? Because you are losing cells, and the actual functional volume of the organ is shrinking. You can have senility in any organ. Unfortunately, one of the biggest risk factors for dementia, and often the earliest sign of dementia risk, is senility in an organ we all know about—the muscles. This form of senility is called sarcopenia, otherwise known as puny and weak muscles.

How can sarcopenia and its under-exercised weak and shrunken muscles be the earliest sign of dementia? Weak muscles indicate we are not exercising. Our muscles are missing the necessary activation process derived from exercise that actually stimulates the brain to grow new memory cells and to repair the current memory cells and the millions of brain synapses that are damaged. There is no question about the connection between strength of muscles and brain stimulation; the research is very clear.[38]

THE IMPORTANCE OF EXERCISE & PHYSICAL ACTIVITY

Having fit muscles is one of the best ways to prevent even the earliest forms of cognitive decline and dementia. Making muscles fitter may also be the most important first step in your *Memory Makeover* program. I'm not saying it is more important than the right diet or optimizing sleep or any of the other strategies that we promote in this book. But it is arguably the easiest step to start if the exercise is initiated gradually and easily, as in taking short walks several times a day.

Exercise includes activities planned into your day that are specifically designed to improve fitness. These activities involve a minimum intensity that would be comparable to a moderately paced walk all the way up to more intensive exercises that make us sweat and get somewhat out of breath. In short, our goal for daily exercise includes participating in walking or something similar that is light to moderate intensity, at least 10 to 15 minutes after each meal.

Additionally, we need to schedule at least 30 to 45 minutes of "get sweaty exercises" every day, including brisk walking, walking hills, jogging, swimming, biking, calisthenics, and anything that gets the heart pumping harder, gets us breathing faster, and feels at least somewhat hard.

Part of this schedule should include muscle-toning exercises at least 2 to 3 times weekly for 20 or more minutes. Remember, this book is just a guide to help you get started in a comprehensive program to optimize brain health. I could write another 300 pages on exercise and there would still be things left unsaid. There are many great resources on this topic.

My main goal here is to emphasize the importance of daily exercise for brain health. Every time we "get sweaty," our brain produces a Brain Derived Neurotrophic Factor (BDNF) that literally heals damaged and dying brain cells. In other words, every day that we don't include some form of exercise we potentially lose hundreds of brain cells that would otherwise have survived if the nourishing and healing effects of BDNF had been activated.

In addition to actual exercise, it is important to be active throughout the day. While planned intense exercise is critical to brain function, simply being mildly active on and off all through the day is of equal importance and equally critical to preventing and reversing cognitive decline. Many of us think that working out for an hour each day is sufficient for health. It's not! If we work out daily but are sitting and inactive the rest of the day, our brains suffer the consequence of our leisure. The research is so strong on this point that "sitting has become the new smoking." Sitting too long each day without intermittent activity is now likely responsible for more cognitive decline than smoking![39] If you exercise daily, you are much less likely to smoke, further lowering your risk for cognitive decline.

We need a daily exercise program, but we also need to be active often throughout the day. Let's look at this in more detail.

PHYSICAL ACTIVITY BATTING AVERAGE

One of the first recommendations I suggest to patients is to assess or review their personal daily Activity Batting Average (ABA). This is like calculating a baseball player's batting average, but in this case comparing the number of hours spent active during the average 24 hours day. To do this, I have them add up how many hours of activity they get in a typical day. I have them include time standing for any reason, doing housework (unless done sitting down), weeding, gardening, working outside, shopping at stores or grocery markets, walking for any reason, walking after meals, riding a bike or swimming, and doing any other form of exercise either at home or at the gym. The sum total of activity time establishes how much of your typical day includes physical activity.

The main benefit of this activity assessment is to realize how much or how little of the day we are actually moving our bodies in a way that increases blood circulation to the brain and stimulates the brain through neuromuscular activation.

The activity time is then compared to hours of the 24-hour day spent as sedentary time. This is the "down time," or time we spend sleeping, sitting, or otherwise not moving or standing.

The main purpose of this evaluation is to show my patients that there is a lot of room for improvement. Even someone who works out at the gym every night for one hour but tends to sit at a desk, on a couch, or at a table the rest of the day ends up with a miserable 24-hour activity average of 4.2%. He or she is therefore active only 4.2% of the day. This is a very poor Activity Batting Average of only 42. Said another way, this person thinks he is doing well but is actually inactive almost 95% of the time.

The goal is to be active a minimum of 10% of the day. This actually requires some level of activity or standing for at least two-and-a-half hours every day. The bottom line is that very few of us are even close to this minimum, even if we work out regularly. But minimum effort does not give maximum benefit. If we want to maximize the brain healing benefit of physical activity, we should aim to gradually increase our activity average into the 20% and then the 30% range. This means making plans so that we are at least standing or moving our body, even if ever so slowly, for 5 to 8 hours each day.

Several generations ago, the average person was at least somewhat active for more than eight hours each day, giving them an activity average of 33 percent. In baseball terms, this would be considered a Batting Average of .330 and referred to as Three Hundred and Thirty or "330." When optimizing brain health with exercise and activity, an optimal activity batting average would be somewhere in the 300 range, but everyone should shoot for a minimum activity average of 10 percent, making your Activity Batting Average (ABA) 100. All this requires is that you avoid sitting down and be active for at least two-and-a-half hours every day!

Just so we aren't tempted to think this is excessive, many who were born before the 1950s remember times when average people were actively standing, walking, or doing something physical up to 12 hours on most days. This gave them an Activity Average of 50 percent (ABA of 500), thus greatly reducing risk of chronic disease and cognitive decline. Sadly, Activity Averages like 50 percent, 33 percent, or even 10 percent are rare these days, and therefore the preventive and curative benefit of activity is typically under-utilized.

But how do we reach a daily Activity Average of 20 to 30 percent involving actively standing or moving for 5 to 8 hours each day? While this may sound utterly absurd, it is actually not that hard to do if you are willing to try.

First of all, we learned elsewhere that light to moderate physical activity immediately after each meal is one of the best strategies to improve brain function. If you go for a 10- to 20-minute stroll after each meal, you already have between 30 minutes to an hour of daily activity. Then you add the more intensive 30+ minute daily workout that should include exercises that make you get sweaty, breathe a little harder, and help strengthen the muscles of your legs, buttocks, arms, back, and chest.

The remaining 3 to 6 hours of activity involve just being on your feet and doing things that require standing or moving your body in some way. If you simply refuse to let yourself sit for more than 2 hours in the morning, 2 hours in the afternoon, and 2 hours in the evening, you will reach your goal! This way, several hours of your morning, afternoon, and evening are spent doing something that involves standing or moving your body. If you tend to work at a desk for many hours each day, you may wish to switch to using an adjustable standing desk. You could end up doing all your computer-based work standing at your adjustable desk, and your activity average would skyrocket.

STRONGER LEG MUSCLES, LESS COGNITIVE DECLINE

In a research study entitled "Kicking Back Cognitive Ageing: Leg Power Predicts Cognitive Ageing after 10 Years in older Female Twins" by Claire J. Steves, findings indicated that thigh muscle strength was associated with improved cognitive aging over 10 years in older female twins. Leg muscle strength is related to physical activity. This means flabbiness, or weakness in leg muscle strength correlates with cognitive decline, while stronger leg muscles may indicate less cognitive decline.[iv]

[iv] For a more complete perspective on the place of exercise in any Wellness program, see the chapter on exercise in my book *Hello Healthy* and my WIN! Wellness, Book 1, *Getting Started, Chapter 3, "Just Do It!—Exercise"* pp. 33-49.

If you're not willing to exercise in order to improve your strength, your balance, and your agility, as well as to prevent falls and lower your risk for heart disease or cancer, at least exercise to optimize the healing potential of your brain.

IMPACT OF POOR TEETH ON THE BRAIN

BL developed and implemented a planned, regular, consistent oral hygiene program as her tenth wellness protocol strategy. How many of us actually floss? My wife is a dental hygienist, I should know better. I've read the research too, but somehow I think I'm above the law and that it doesn't really matter whether or not I floss.

The reality, however, is that if you do not floss, you are at greater risk of heart disease, cancer, and Alzheimer's. Why? Because not flossing means you are more likely, depending on many factors, to have inflammatory changes in your mouth that become systemic and spread to the rest of your body. This includes increasing inflammation in the brain, which stimulates excess production of beta amyloid plaques and other factors that fatally damage brain cells and synapses associated with cognitive function and limit access to past memories.

Dental care is often the weakest part of an individual's health plan. People tend to think that daily dental care is all about cosmetics and not ultimately that important to health. The truth is, oral hygiene is critically important to health because, for many people, body-wide inflammation is almost entirely due to gingivitis or periodontal disease. Gingivitis and periodontal disease drive multiple chronic diseases, risk of autoimmunity, and many other inflammatory conditions, including Alzheimer's.[40] So yes, we all need to floss!

IMPACT OF HORMONE REPLACEMENT THERAPY

The 11th strategy BL agreed to was to reinstate appropriate Hormone Replacement Therapy (HRT) as part of her personal neurological wellness protocol. She had stopped hormone therapy in 2002 because the Women's Health Initiative study at that time had created concerns about breast cancer and blood clots. However, there are simple and effective ways to use bioidentical hormone strategies individualized according to clinical need and based on appropriate lab testing.

Multiple hormones directly influence the brain's ability to protect, heal, and even grow new cells, as well as to support the synaptic connections between neurons. For instance, it has been said that estrogen is to memory for women what testosterone is to memory for men.

Additionally, thyroid hormone balance is critically important for cognitive function.[41] Having even slightly low levels of thyroid hormones associated with hypothyroidism can be a significant trigger for declining memory and brain function over time.

Other hormones like DHEA, progesterone, and pregnenolone have been associated with protection of the brain. [42] Having optimal levels of these hormones is associated with less buildup of the destructive beta amyloid plaques found in Alzheimer's Disease[43].

If laboratory testing determines that one or more of these hormones are at suboptimal levels, appropriately supplementing them could limit the risk or progression of Alzheimer's and greatly enhance potential for reversing various symptoms of cognitive decline. But merely supplementing these hormones to optimize blood levels isn't good enough. The first and most important step in balancing hormones has to do with following a comprehensive lifestyle medicine approach.

This includes putting a priority on exercise, a whole plant-based diet, stress management, and making sure your home and work environments are not exposing you to toxins from smoking, pesticides, bacteria, fungi, viruses, and mold biotoxins.

IMPACT OF 12-HOUR FAST

BL implemented a 12-hour intermittent fast every evening between dinner and breakfast for her twelfth wellness protocol strategy. This is a powerful strategy for improving many facets of health. A 12-hour intermittent fast means that once you finish your evening meal (preferably before 7 o'clock), you don't put another morsel of food in your mouth (or any other form of calories) until breakfast the next morning.

Avoiding all calories for extended times is beneficial to health, but low blood sugar tendencies should be addressed and corrected prior to initiating an extended intermittent fast. This can be most effectively assessed by doing a 4-hour Glucose tolerance test. If someone is having a hypoglycemic reaction for whatever reason, perhaps because of using or producing excess insulin, then food must be taken to bring the blood sugar back up to a normal level. If your blood sugar is crashing to a low level, it is imperative to fix the problem promptly. You may need to work up to the point where you can effectively go without food for 12 or more hours. For many of us, an 18-hour fast involving only two meals daily might be even better.

It is important to understand that having low blood sugar (hypoglycemia) is extremely detrimental to your brain. High blood sugar is very bad for your brain as well, but low blood sugar is even worse. High blood sugars are not only damaging or toxic to brain cells, but the very nature of high blood sugar means you may not be getting the needed sugar into your brain cells, thus causing many of them to die from lack of energy support.

Having optimal blood sugar is necessary for proper brain function and especially for maintaining functional memory. Interestingly, we cannot make memories unless our blood sugar is high enough. But more importantly, we cannot make a memory last more than a few minutes unless the sugar is actually getting into the neurons of the hippocampus. Further, even when the sugar is adequate in our brain's blood stream, that sugar is not going to do us any good without adequate insulin needed to store the sugar in the brain cell.

In countless animal studies, researchers have found that giving a healthy animal a little dose of insulin enables the animal to memorize a maze more quickly. Thus, we know that insulin in of itself is not bad; what is bad is when your body becomes insulin resistant. A certain level of insulin should be adequate to help you store sugar in your brain cells. But if your brain cells are resistant to insulin, it will take a lot more insulin to actually store sugar in the neurons and make and retain memories.

One of the best ways to measure this is with a specialized FDG PET scan using fluoro-deoxy-glucose. This form of glucose can be traced by the PET scan, allowing the doctor to determine whether the brain cells are actually absorbing and metabolically using the glucose. If the sugar is not getting into the brain, this is called hypometabolism, in which case the brain (or at least a certain region of the brain) is insulin resistant. This is a key component of Alzheimer's. However, this FDG PET scan costs thousands of dollars and is typically not covered by insurance for evaluating cognitive decline.

In my opinion, the most functional blood test for evaluating insulin resistance is to do a 4-hour Glucose tolerance test that checks both glucose and insulin blood levels after ingesting 75 grams of glucose in a sugary carbonated drink at the lab. Having elevated blood sugars anytime during this test is a strong sign of insulin resistance. This typically stimulates the pancreas to produce large amounts of insulin, thus creating even more problems for the brain, including hypoglycemia one to three hours later. This roller coaster of high and low sugars limits our ability to properly transfer short-term memories into long term memory.[v]

So how is the 12- to 18-hour fast beneficial? If I find myself gaining an extra roll of fat in my midsection, which I do from time to time, I should consider extending the 12 hours to 18. When this happens, I say to myself, "Wes, you don't need to eat dinner tonight because your body can feast on this tummy all night long." Certainly there is plenty of energy there. I just accept the fact that for the next week—or two or three—I've got to get myself back into gear. As my own decision maker, I know I don't need that third meal of the day. I eat breakfast, a good lunch, and then I go on my 18-hour intermittent fast.

What happens to your body when you do this? Your body becomes more effective and efficient at burning fat, which of course is the entire goal. Your body much more effectively burns the food up that you consume for breakfast and lunch than any food you eat in the afternoon or evening. The result is a significant increase in your

---

[v] For further explanation of "insulin resistance" see *Goodbye Diabetes*, by Dr. Wes Youngberg, pp. 21, 22, 271, 272. Available winwellness.org and dryoungberg.com.

metabolism. More importantly, studies have documented that intermittent fasting initiates a mild ketosis that can help naturally repair hippocampal memory defects and promote the growth of new memory neurons—a process called neurogenesis.[44][45][46][vi]

FACTORS THAT YIELD INCREDIBLE RESULTS

Let's take a minute and review exactly what BL did to change her lifestyle and her health care program. These were the actions she took for her personalized wellness protocol.

1. Eliminate simple carbohydrates.
2. Eliminate all processed foods.
3. Eliminate gluten.
4. Increase vegetable and fruit intake.
5. Implement stress reduction.
6. Increase sleep to 7 to 8 hours per night.
7. Use 1,000 micrograms of vitamin B12 daily.
8. Use 2,000 international units of vitamin D3 daily.
9. Exercise for 30 minutes 4 to 6 times per week.
10. Practice oral hygiene consistently.
11. Use Hormone Replacement Therapy.
12. Observe an intermittent 12-hour fast each day.

[vi] For a discussion on mealtime—when and how often—see chapter 4, "It's a Gut Feeling," pp. 91-92, in *Hello Healthy,* by Dr. Wes Youngberg, available at winwellness.org or dryoungberg.com

In order to arrive at a personalized list of recommended strategies for my patients, I routinely spend several sessions discussing the patient's personal and family medical history and reviewing labs and reports from previous years. This review determines which additional labs need to be done.

At the first visit, I encourage the patient to order the *23andme.com* saliva genetic test, which takes up to one month to process. For a general background on the place of genes in a wellness program, see chapter 12, "But I've Got Bad Genes," in *Pressing Forward,* book 2 of my WIN! Wellness series. Also see chapter 1, "Are There Holes in Your Genes? Reaching Your Full Genetic Potential," in my book *Hello Healthy: Strategies to Reach your Full Health and Wellness Potential.*

INCREDIBLE CHANGES WITHIN THREE MONTHS

BL's protocol represents potentially huge lifestyle changes. You might ask, "How long did it take for BL's brain to start working properly again?"

Great question! It took only three months!

For some reason, we mistakenly believe that once the brain has a problem, then the brain is always going to have that problem. Do we really think the God, who is our loving Father, made the most important, most complex organ in the universe, the human brain, so that it couldn't heal? I don't believe that for a nanosecond. I do think the more important question is, "What do I need to change now in my lifestyle in order to improve my brain function?"

Also, realize that this was not a three-month period where BL said, "Well, I think today I'll have just one piece of cake. What could it hurt?" Or "I'm busy today so I'll just try to exercise tomorrow," Or "Yesterday's walk did not really seem to help me, so maybe I can skip it every so often." Or "Today, I should try taking some vitamin D," then after a week or so thinking, "Well, I've heard that vitamin D can be toxic at high doses, and I'd rather not take supplements, so I'm going to stop taking it daily as suggested."

Second guessing the protocol as outlined by your functional and lifestyle medicine specialist is not only unwise, but it will likely undermine the potential effectiveness of the program. If a friend or even another health professional questions what you are doing, discuss this with your specialist before making any changes to your personal wellness protocol.

When it comes to improving brain function, and especially when seeking to reverse symptoms of cognitive decline, it is imperative to address your multiple risk factors collectively and at the same time. By doing this, your brain has the best opportunity to start healing. It will not be effective to do just little baby steps here and there, now and then; you have to address all the factors contributing to the problems and consistently implement them over time.

CHAPTER 12

ENTREPRENEUR:
BREDESEN CASE STUDY

OUR NEXT CASE STUDY ALSO COMES from Dr. Bredesen's 2014 paper.[47] It involves a 69-year-old male entrepreneur (ETP).

For the last 11 years, ETP had been experiencing progressive memory loss. At the age of 58, he was unable to recall the locker combination at his health club, and he thought, "Wow! That is really weird. I've been coming here for so many years. How could I forget?"

ETP was a successful businessman, yet he couldn't remember the simple combination to his locker. This reality gave ETP cause for pause. He decided to talk to his doctor about the concern.

TESTING USED TO DETERMINE RISK

First, a FDG PET imaging scan was completed, and the results indicated early Alzheimer's patterns with reduced glucose utilization by brain cells. The results from this PET scan were critical to understanding the underlying problem ETP was experiencing, because one way that Alzheimer's can be diagnosed in its early stages is to discover how well the brain can actually take in sugar from the blood into its neurons for energy production.

When the brain is not able to properly utilize or take in sugar from the blood, this is referred to as insulin resistance of the brain. Researchers refer to this as type 3 diabetes, or as diabetes of the brain. Thus, the concepts discussed in the treatment process and the interventions used are very similar to the methods used in reversing insulin resistance of the body (typically of the liver and muscle cells), as experienced in metabolic syndrome, prediabetes, and type 2 diabetes.

Understanding the implications of this is important, as I will more clearly demonstrate later.

HOPE BEYOND DIP IN VERBAL LEARNING TEST SCORES

At the age of 58, ETP completed the California Verbal Learning Test (CVLT) and scored in the 84th percentile. These results indicated that ETP had a higher verbal learning score than 84 percent of U.S. adults.

Over the next 11-years, ETP's score declined all the way down to the 1st percentile. This meant that in one decade, ETP dropped from being in the top 16 percent of the nation to being in the bottom 1 percent; meaning that at that point 99 percent of all American adults had better brain function than ETP.

While reviewing his genetic report with his doctor, ETP learned that, along with 70 million Americans or essentially 25 percent of the population, he had a single copy mutation of ApoE4—the Alzheimer's gene.

Having the ApoE4 mutation instead of the normal ApoE3 non-mutated gene doubles the risk of cardiovascular disease and exponentially increases the risk of Alzheimer's. From a genetic perspective, the ApoE4 gene mutation represents a greater risk than all the other Alzheimer's related gene mutations combined. The healthy ApoE3 gene provides codes for the production of protein molecules that help break down and remove the beta amyloid plaques that are toxic to brain cells and associated with Alzheimer's.

Each of us has one copy of the ApoE gene from each parent. If one parent gives us a normal copy of ApoE and our other parent gives us the mutated copy of ApoE, we end up with an ApoE3/E4 combination. This combination statistically increases our risk of Alzheimer's an average of 2- to 5-fold. If both parents give us a mutated copy, we end up with a double copy mutation represented as ApoE4/E4, which is associated with a dramatic 5- to 34-fold increase in risk of Alzheimer's. Study reviews suggest that the average or typical increase in risk is 12-fold.

It is important to note that up to 50 percent of those who develop Alzheimer's do not carry this APoE4 gene mutation. Other factors and genes also impact this risk. Thankfully, there are ways to neutralize and manage these genetic risk factors, which are largely reversible, with broad-based, anti-inflammatory strategies.

In addition, we all have other gene mutations that influence Alzheimer's risk to some degree. Specifically, each of us who thoroughly reviews our genetic reports with an experienced specialist will discover many other genes with double copy mutations and some with single copies.

ETP needed to evaluate those other risk factors with blood testing. The key here was to optimize every area of health. This would include addressing and optimizing digestion, detoxification, low-grade infections, elevated cardiac CRP, and other forms of inflammation.

At this point, ETP had not worked with a specialist that could guide him in developing an individualized personal wellness protocol. He became progressively unable to recognize faces at work. He required a full-time assistant to prompt and guide every task. The lifetime ability ETP possessed, adding columns of numbers rapidly in his head, was lost. This was of great concern since the skill was needed for his profession. Thus, ETP's effectiveness at work was dramatically decreasing.

ETP completed the recommended blood tests and discovered his homocysteine was extremely high at 18 micromol/L; the level should be between 6 and 8. His cardiac CRP, also known as high sensitivity CRP, a measure of inflammation, was actually perfect.

This indicates the need to be very careful in determining health risk based solely on one test. Just because this very helpful measure of systemic inflammation is optimal, (less than 0.5), one cannot be certain that there are no indications of inflammation. The results did mean that ETP did not have that specific form of inflammation as measured by the CRP test.

I have seen patients who have an extremely high level of inflammation based on the sedimentation rate and yet a very low level of inflammation based on the CRP test and vice versa. For this reason, it is wise to test broadly. Step back and look at the entire mosaic of risk factors; do not make decisions based on the results of just one test, as this can be very misleading.

Normal or Optimal

Dr. Bredesen emphasized a key concept of an effective protocol in his 2014 UCLA paper published in the journal *Aging*. Do not be satisfied, he cautioned, when lab tests are found to be within the normal reference range. A reference range is typically defined as the set of values that include 95 percent of the general population. This is also known as the 95 percent prediction interval.[48] In other words, for most lab tests, unless your lab value is smaller than the lowest 2.5 percent of the general population or larger than the highest 2.5 percent of the population, you are considered to have a "normal" lab value.

I do not have a problem with calling these statistical ranges "normal," but they certainly aren't healthy, nor are they anywhere near optimal. Normal should never be associated with optimal health. As an example, 67 percent of the U.S. population is overweight, and most of them would fit within the statistical definition of normal. Since nearly 50 percent of adults over age 40 have prediabetes, they would also be called "normal."

A 2019 health statistics update from the American Heart Association reports that 48 percent of adults in the U.S. currently have cardiovascular disease.[49] It is therefore statistically "normal" to have heart disease. And since nearly half of adults 85 and older have Alzheimer's, it is also statistically "normal" to have Alzheimer's.

Normal lab ranges simply represent the *typical* health of the population. I'm pretty certain than no one reading this book has any interest in a normal progression of ill health. By challenging ourselves to optimize every lab test, we have a chance to rise above the mediocrity of "normal" health and thus prevent and potentially reverse our "normal" symptoms of cognitive decline.

For instance, we know that the high blood levels of insulin, cardiac CRP, lipoproteine(a), and homocysteine, to name a few, are much more significant risk factors for heart disease and for Alzheimer's than is a high cholesterol. And yet a high cholesterol is still an important predictor of risk and should be addressed.

But did you know that prior to 1984 the "normal" lab reference ranges for cholesterol were between 130 and 320? The ranges were based on the above statistical model that assumes 95 percent of the population is normal and therefore are considered in the acceptable range.

That's right! Back then, if your doctor checked your cholesterol and it was 310, he or she would have told you that your cholesterol was normal, and no diet or drug treatment would have been prescribed. It was only after statin medications became available in the mid 1980s that new clinical ranges were established recommending cholesterol levels less than 200. This was based on what experts reported to be a more clinically optimal reference range associated with much lower risk for cardiovascular disease.

As we begin to assess our health risk factors, our main goal is to highlight every lab or finding that is not currently in the optimal range. Of course, this requires working with a health care team and/or specialist who understands optimal labs values for each test and also practices optimal individualized strategies for achieving optimal reversal of cognitive decline.

IMPACT OF VITAMINS AND HORMONES LEVELS

ETP's vitamin D level was low at 28 ng/ml,—not super low, but definitely deficient. Many studies indicate that vitamin D levels need to be above 50. I personally believe that the most protective vitamin D blood level is somewhere between 60 and 100 ng/ml. Unless already supplementing vitamin D daily, my experience is that most of my patients find their vitamin D levels to be very suboptimal somewhere between 20 and 35 ng/ml. Typically, I recommend taking a minimum of 5,000 to 10,000 IUs daily and then rechecking blood levels in three to six months in order to make individualized adjustments in their daily dose.[vii]

ETP's hormone pregnenolone level was very low; pregnenolone is the master hormone that is enzymatically converted directly from cholesterol. The way you get an adequate level of pregnenolone is by having an adequate level of cholesterol. Cholesterol is not bad in of itself; God designed every cell of your body with the capacity to make its own cholesterol. It is a critical part of building the structure of every cell; cholesterol is also essential in the production of vitamin D as well as of many hormones in the body.

ETP's serum copper to zinc ratio was very imbalanced. There exists a substantial amount of medical research on the relationship between zinc, copper, and Alzheimer's.[50][51] The information is throughout the medical literature. In fact, the copper/zinc nutrient ratio balance is also an indicator of risk for cardiovascular disease as well as other health concerns.

[vii] For more information on vitamin D testing and interpreting the results of the 25(OH)D test, see WIN! Wellness, Book 1, *Getting Started,* pp. 54-55. The books *Hello Healthy* and *Goodbye Diabetes* also have chapters on vitamin D.

PERSONALIZED WELLNESS PROTOCOL

Below are the key elements of ETP's personalized wellness protocol, an individualized lifestyle program implemented as a result of proper diagnosis and testing. You will recognize that some elements of the protocol are the same as BL's. Others that are specific to ETP's choices are further discussed below.

1. Fast (no food) for at least 3 hours before bedtime, which is very important for improving sleep.
2. Observe 12 hours of intermittent fasting every day.
3. Eliminate all simple carbohydrates.
4. Eliminate all processed foods.
5. Eliminate meats and fish unless organic.
6. Use probiotics daily to improve digestive health.
7. Increase vegetable and fruit intake.
8. Exercise strenuously.
9. Use individualized supplements daily.

ROLE OF DIGESTION IN REVERSING MENTAL DECLINE

There is a huge relationship between the microbiome, the gut, and the brain. In addition to approximately 20,000 genes in the human body, the body is host to trillions of cells, including bacteria and fungi, many of which are beneficial. Most of them reside in the gut.
Collectively they are known as the microbiome, "an ecosystem of microorganisms that inhabit a particular environment in or on the human body. Our gut microbiome consists of tens of trillions of microorganisms

such as bacteria, fungi, and viruses. They help us digest our food, regulate our immune system, protect against other bacteria that cause disease, and produce vitamins. They are also important in the maintenance of normal and healthy brain function."[52]

Johns Hopkins University is conducting amazing research focused on the relationship between the gut and the brain. Dr. Jay Pasricha, director for the Center for Neurogastroenterology, states, "We now have proof that, not only do they [intestinal nerve cells] regenerate, but the whole network turns completely over every few weeks in adult animals." This research further documents that new nerve cells are born daily all throughout our body, but especially in our gut and brain.

"After the brain, the digestive tract contains the largest nervous system in the human body."[53] In other words, how well we treat our digestive system greatly determines our potential to optimize and heal the brain.

A healthy digestive system also translates to a healthy immune function. We now know that at least 70 percent of our entire immune system resides in the gut. This relationship also extends to the lymphatic system. Pure and simple, if we don't have a healthy gut, we are not going to have a healthy brain.

This is a prime reason why we must "fix" digestion. Poor digestion is not just an inconvenience or perhaps an embarrassment in social situations. Digestion is a critical part of the body's healing system and, if not working properly, we will not heal properly. That includes healing and ultimately brain functionality. If you have any concerns about digestion, make sure to read the entire chapter, "It's a Gut Feeling: Optimizing Digestion," in my book *Hello Healthy*. My book *Goodbye Diabetes* also has a 19-

page chapter on how to naturally address bloating, reflux, and other digestive concerns.

EXERCISE AND SLEEP IN WELLNESS PROTOCOL

Why is strenuous exercise valuable to health and healing? The word "strenuous" can be interpreted in many ways. I tell my patients that healthy, strenuous exercise for them is when they feel like the exercise is "somewhat hard" and they are a little out of breath but can still talk to their workout partner while exercising. If they can whistle while exercising, then it is not appropriately strenuous.

Aim to strenuously exercise at least three but preferably five or more times per week—for example, swimming, cycling, running. Don't forget to do strength-training exercises like weights or simple calisthenics at least twice weekly as well.

In our case study, ETP was very motivated. He was determined to heal his brain. He also increased his sleep to 7 or 8 hours per night. He wasn't 100 percent successful in changing his sleep patterns, but he did what he could.

SUPPLEMENTS USED

ETP took melatonin to support the brain healing qualities of sleep. He also took enough vitamin B12, methyl folate, and vitamin B6 to lower his elevated blood homocysteine levels.

Working closely with his doctor, ETP started taking appropriate doses of three different herbs: bacopa monnieri, ashwaganda, and turmeric. Additionally, ETP used citicoline (also known as CDP Choline), which is well documented in medical journals to improve cognitive function in patients with cognitive impairment.[54] All four nutritional supplements support brain health.

Like most people, ETP had no idea that his brain was also at risk because of inadequate levels of vitamin D in his blood. ETP figured that if vitamin D was that important, his physician would have ordered a test years ago. Because of his many years of significant cognitive decline, ETP sought out a doctor who was much more proactive about discovering every modifiable risk factor for dementia and then recommending strategies to fix each one.

Testing for and optimizing his vitamin D level was one of the simplest fixes in the entire program. All ETP needed to do was take 5,000 IUs of vitamin D3 daily and then retest after 3 to 6 months to ensure he was on the right dose.

Meeting regularly with his specialist, ETP requested guidance on which herbs and supplements were most likely to provide additional neurotrophic support. A neurotrophic substance enhances cognition and memory and facilitates learning. After reviewing ETP's medical chart more closely and considering his list of risk factors and symptoms, they decided to move forward with three herbs that have substantial research support for their neurotrophic benefits and safety. ETP started taking bacopa monnieri at 250mg once daily; ashwaganda at 500 mg once daily; and turmeric at 400 mg daily. But just because these herbs and doses were used by ETP and are often used by my patients with cognitive concerns doesn't mean that they are the right herbs and doses for everyone. Each of us must establish an individualized list of neurotrophic support supplements based on our own medical history, our goals, and the combination of our risk factors that need to be addressed.

BENEFITS OF ASHWAGANDHA

There is more than adequate scientific support and peer-reviewed, evidence-based papers on the judicious use of ashwagandha, bacopa, and turmeric for dementia.[55] One scientific review published in the journal *Alzheimer's Research and Therapy* states in its abstract, "This review gathers research on various medicinal plants that have shown promise in reversing the Alzheimer's disease pathology."[56] Not only do the reports give credence to the use of these herbs, but even Dr. Rudolph Tanzi, a celebrated professor of neurology at Harvard University School of Medicine, has documented the benefits of ashwagandha root extract, stating that it "has been shown to help export the plaque out of the brain."[57] [58]

Dr. Tanzi is a likeable and gracious man who also is personally responsible for discovering the majority of the genes associated with Alzheimer's disease. As a sought-after speaker at medical conferences, he often describes in great detail how ashwagandha helps remove toxic oxidized beta amyloid plaques from the brain. He also practices what he preaches by taking 500 mg of ashwagandha root extract once daily.

BENEFITS OF TURMERIC AND CURCUMIN

Turmeric and its active ingredient curcumin appear to have even broader therapeutic benefits than ashwagandha. I personally use 800 mg of a 95 percent standardized curcumin supplement daily. It has so many clinical applications that I recommend its use to many of my patients and practically to every patient who is interested in preventing or reversing cognitive decline.

As an example of the many studies and reports supporting the use of curcumin, here is an abstract from a 2018 paper, "Use of curcumin in diagnosis, prevention, and treatment of Alzheimer's disease," published in the journal *Neural Regeneration Research*:

"This review summarizes and describes the use of curcumin in diagnosis, prevention, and treatment of Alzheimer's disease. For diagnosis of Alzheimer's disease, amyloid-β and highly phosphorylated tau protein are the major biomarkers. Curcumin was developed as an early diagnostic probe based on its natural fluorescence and high binding affinity to amyloid-β. Because of its multi-target effects, curcumin has protective and preventive effects on many chronic diseases such as cerebrovascular disease, hypertension, and hyperlipidemia. For prevention and treatment of Alzheimer's disease, curcumin has been shown to effectively maintain the normal structure and function of cerebral vessels, mitochondria, and synapses, reduce risk factors for a variety of chronic diseases, and decrease the risk of Alzheimer's disease. The effect of curcumin on Alzheimer's disease involves multiple signaling pathways: anti-amyloid and metal iron chelating properties, antioxidation and anti-inflammatory activities. Indeed, there is a scientific basis for the rational application of curcumin in prevention and treatment of Alzheimer's disease."[59]

BENEFITS OF BACOPA

A 1996 study presented at the International Brain Research Conference indicated that bacopa could cut the time required for learning a new task in half. A rigorous 2001 study involving a double-blind, randomized, placebo-

120

controlled experiment conducted in Portland, Oregon, by professors of four different universities, showed that elderly subjects "scored higher on cognitive processing tests after 12 weeks" of taking 300 mg of bacopa once daily. [60] The study included 54 participants whose average age was 73 years. Of interest was that bacopa improved cognitive function in these participants even though none of them had clinical signs of dementia.

These results were substantiated by a study out of the University of Wollongong in Australia's psychology department, which indicated that taking bacopa substantially increases both memory and recall.[61] This was a double blind, placebo-controlled study including 76 adults, ages 40 to 65. Taking 300 mg of bacopa once daily for three months led to significant improvement in the retention of new information. "Follow-up tests showed that the rate of learning was unaffected, suggesting that Brahmi [bacopa] decreases the rate of forgetting of newly acquired information."[62]

Researchers have "conducted hundreds of studies examining the mechanisms of action [of bacopa] on the brain and at a cellular level. Interestingly this research has uncovered a myriad of possible mechanisms relating to anti-inflammatory, antioxidant, metal chelation, amyloid, and cholinergic effects amongst many others. Although it is not unusual for plant-based medicines to have multiple effects on cellular processes, Bacopa Monnieri is perhaps one of the most scientifically studied substances in terms of mechanisms of action. Interestingly, these mechanisms seem to comprehensively map on to the biological mechanisms that many researchers have argued underpin cognitive and memory processes."[63]

While research continues to guide our decisions on what strategies are most effective and safe, it is reasonable to expect, based on the many studies done to date, that the use of bacopa, as researched at 300 mg once daily, can be one of our many proactive strategies to slow down, stop, and even potentially reverse various aspects of cognitive decline. It is important to note that any new medicine, vitamin, food, or beverage has the potential to have negative side effects, especially when first used. To better understand potential side effects of normally beneficial herbs, I often consult Dr. Andrew Weil's website at *DrWeil.com.*

Combining a Harvard education and a lifetime of practicing natural and preventive medicine, Dr. Weil is the founder and director of the Arizona Center for Integrative Medicine at the University of Arizona, where he also holds the Lovell-Jones endowed chair in integrative rheumatology and is clinical professor of medicine and professor of public health.[64]

This is what Dr. Weil reports with regard to bacopa, "For memory and cognition, 300 mg of bacopa extract per day for 12 weeks was found to be safe and effective. Used as recommended, bacopa is generally considered safe. Side effects may include nausea, dry mouth, and fatigue."

If you try bacopa and experience a significant level of either of these side effects, then maybe this herb isn't right for you. Remember, while the average person does very well with bacopa, that doesn't mean it should be on your priority list.

So now we know about many of the strategies specifically used by ETP. But what were the results? After 11 years of progressive memory and cognitive loss had all his efforts actually benefited him?

Let's review the very words Dr. Bredesen used in reporting ETP's results as documented in the 2016 paper, "Reversal of cognitive decline in Alzheimer's disease."

Before starting his personalized wellness protocol, ETP "noted that he had progressive difficulty recognizing the faces at work (prosopagnosia), and had to have his assistants prompt him with the daily schedule. He also recalled an event during which he was several chapters into a book before he finally realized that it was a book he had read previously. In addition, he lost an ability he had had for most of his life: the ability to add columns of numbers rapidly in his head. He was advised that, given his status as an Alzheimer's disease patient and his clear progression, as well as his poor performance on the 2013 test, he should begin to 'get his affairs in order.' His business was in the process of being shut down due to his inability to continue work....

"[A]fter six months [of carefully following his personalized wellness protocol as outlined above], his wife, co-workers, and he all noted improvement. He lost 10 pounds. He was able to recognize faces at work unlike before, was able to remember his daily schedule, and was able to function at work without difficulty. He was also noted to be quicker with his responses. His life-long ability to add columns of numbers rapidly in his head, which he had lost during his progressive cognitive decline, returned. His wife pointed out that, although he had clearly shown improvement, the more striking effect was that he had been accelerating in his decline over the prior year or two, and this had been completely halted.

"After 22 months on the program, he returned for follow-up quantitative neuropsychological testing, which revealed marked improvement: his CVLT-IIB had increased from 3rd percentile to 84th percentile (3 standard deviations), total recognized hits from <1st percentile to 50th percentile, CVLT-II from 54th percentile to 96th percentile, auditory delayed memory from 13th percentile to 79th percentile, reverse digit span from 24th percentile to 74th percentile, and processing speed from 93rd percentile to 98th percentile. His business, which had been in the process of termination, was reinvigorated, and a new site was added to the previous sites of operation."

In closing his report, Dr. Bredesen further commented, "This patient had well-documented Alzheimer's disease, with an ApoE4-positive genotype, characteristic FDG-PET scan, characteristic abnormalities on neuropsychological testing, well documented decline on longitudinal quantitative neuropsychological testing, and progression of symptoms. After two years on the protocol, his symptoms and neuropsychological testing improved markedly. The neuropsychologist who performed and evaluated his testing pointed out that his improvement was beyond that which had been observed in the neuropsychologist's 30 years of practice."

Many of us remember Cher's amazing comeback single "If I Could Turn Back Time." In 1989, after years of scandals and challenges in her personal life, Cher captured the nostalgic pulse of a generation that was full of regrets. Regardless of what you think about Cher, the lyrics of that song cut deep into the emotional foundation of our hopes and dreams. Too often those emotions are just brushed aside as if they represent hopes that are gone forever. What ETP had discovered is that he could turn back time. He had in fact found a way!

Isn't this powerful! Can you imagine turning back 11 years of mental decline in just *six months* and then continuing to improve year to year? ETP is one more example of what is possible. There is indeed hope for us all.

CHAPTER 13

NOTHING SO POWERFUL AS THE TRUTH

SIR WINSTON CHURCHILL ONCE SAID, "Men stumble over the truth from time to time, but most pick themselves up and hurry off as if nothing happened." When John stumbled across the potential to prevent further cognitive decline in Mary and possibly even reverse portions of her dementia, he did not make the all too common mistake of wistfully dismissing it as wishful thinking. He didn't fall into the trap of assuming, like many others in similar circumstances, that if it were really true their doctor would have recommended it.

After brief consideration of the protocol, many simply move on to the next story on the Internet. They pick themselves up and hurry off as if nothing has happened. In doing so, they inadvertently miss one of the most important opportunities for healing.

Dr. E. William Rosenberg, MD, is credited as saying, "It is very unscientific to not have an open mind." John was fortunate to have an open-minded neurologist who paid more attention to the *science and art* of healing than he did to the *convention and politics* of healing.

American orator and politician Daniel Webster wrote, "There is nothing so powerful as truth." Expanding on this, Jim Collins, in his book *Good to Great,* stated, "There is a sense of exhilaration that comes from facing head-on the hard Truths, and saying, 'We will never give up. We will never capitulate. It might take a long time, but we will find a way to prevail.'" John and Mary had found "the road less traveled." They had found a way and had prevailed. They would never give up, nor would they ever capitulate.

THINKING LOGICALLY ABOUT TREATMENT OF COGNITIVE DECLINE

C. S. Lewis is one of my favorite authors. He was raised by a mother who graduated from Queens College with First Class Honors in logic.[65] The discipline of properly using logic to distinguish truth from error was powerfully instilled in him. He effectively used it all his life, which is evident in his writings.

It never ceases to amaze me how even intelligent people often show an inability to think logically. They may have a keen memory, being able to quickly remember hundreds of protocols learned as students for treating various health conditions, but when asked how their treatments actually address the multiple underlying causes of disease, they are without a good answer.

"I simply follow the clinical guidelines considered to be the current standard of care," they often say. Highly educated doctors who are board certified in their specialties have at times said to me that there is no evidence that the cognitive decline of Alzheimer's can be reversed. In my view, they can only make this statement from ignorance and/or an unwillingness to explore the vast amount of evidence that is already in the medical literature.

It's much like saying that there is no evidence that Guam exists, because few people who grew up elsewhere have ever been to Guam. Therefore, they choose to believe that it doesn't exist, in part because they have never seen it for themselves. It's a silly analogy, but it's also silly and illogical to say that something can't be done when people all over the world, provided with the right clinical direction, have in fact done just that. Not just one person but many people have done it, and the results continue to be published in peer-reviewed medical journals.

100 CASES OF REVERSAL

While this concise how-to guide includes just a few case studies as examples and demonstrations of what is possible and how it is done, there is much more proof elsewhere. One hundred examples can be found in a 2018 paper published in the *Journal of Alzheimer's Disease & Parkinsonism.* In this paper, Dr. Dale Bredesen, myself, and 21 other doctors collectively presented our case studies showing reversal of cognitive decline in 100 of our current patients.[66]

"THE ROAD LESS TRAVELED BY"

The controversy of whether symptoms of cognitive decline can be reversed or even prevented reminds me of a classic poem written by Edgar A. Guest entitled, "It Couldn't Be Done."

Somebody said that it couldn't be done,
  But he with a chuckle replied
That 'maybe it couldn't' but he would be one
  Who wouldn't say so till he'd tried.

So he buckled right in with the trace of a grin
  On his face. If he worried he hid it.
He started to sing as he tackled the thing
  That couldn't be done, and he did it. . .

"There are thousands to tell you it cannot be done,
  There are thousands to prophesy failure;
There are thousands to point out to you, one by one,
  The dangers that wait to assail you.

But just buckle in with a bit of a grin,
  Just take off your coat and go to it;
Just start to sing as you tackle the thing
  That 'cannot be done,' and you'll do it.

A poem by Robert Frost speaks of the road "less traveled by, and that has made all the difference." Regardless of Frost's original meaning, these words conjure up a perceived truth. We cannot let ourselves be overly influenced by conventional opinion. To succeed in life, we must rise above the mediocre expectations of others and take that "road less traveled by." Doing that will make all the difference.

Two roads diverged in a wood, and I—
I took the one less traveled by,
And that has made all the difference.

RESOURCES

The **Diabetes Undone Kit** focuses on helping patients fully reverse insulin resistance. It is typically the first resource I recommend to my patients because insulin resistance is the most common trigger of cognitive decline. The kit includes a full workbook, journal, meal plan, and a plant-based cookbook. The best part of the kit is the 40 short, 7- to 10-minute videos where I walk the viewer through the steps to fully reverse insulin resistance as well as the foundational lifestyle medicine strategies associated with starting a personal wellness protocol. Ten of the videos feature internationally acclaimed nutritionist Brenda Davis, RD. Together, we discuss how to effectively use a plant-strong diet to reverse chronic disease.
Available at dryoungberg.com.

My book **Hello Healthy: Strategies to Reach Your Full Health and Wellness Potential** provides the best overview of what patients need to know to get healthy again. It is typically the first book I recommend that my patients read in order to optimize the effectiveness of our clinical consultations. It also includes a full chapter on epigenetics and a 45-page section explaining the rationale and interpretation of the majority of specialty labs I recommend.
Available at dryoungberg.com and winwellness.org.

The **"12 Weeks to Wellness" DVD series** is the video version of my book *Hello Healthy* and includes twelve 90-minute presentations:

Part 1: Optimizing your Genetic Potential
Part 2: Optimizing your Metabolism
Part 3: Optimizing Circulation and Heart Health
Part 4: Sunlight, vitamin D, and Health
Part 5: Optimizing Digestion for Health and Healing
Part 6: Stress, Emotions, Food, Adrenals, Caffeine, and Blood Sugars
Part 7: Attitudes and Health Risk
Part 8: Preventing and Reversing Chronic Kidney Disease
Part 9: The Autoimmune Epidemic—Ways to Limit Your own Risk
Part 10: Detoxification for Optimal Health
Part 11: Sleep and Health-Maximizing your Healing Potential
Part 12: Best Lab Tests for Maximizing your Healing Potential

These video presentations are often used by individual patients to maximize their learning. They can also be used to run group sessions at clinics, churches, community centers, or home-based share groups.
Available at dryoungberg.com and winwellness.org.

Goodbye Diabetes: Preventing and Reversing Diabetes the Natural Way is my comprehensive lifestyle medicine book for reversing insulin resistance, which is the key driver of most chronic diseases including cardiovascular disease, diabetes, cancer and neurocognitive disorders leading to Alzheimer's.
Available at dryoungberg.com and winwellness.org.

WIN! Wellness "On The Path To Health and Healing" is a series I was privileged to co-author with my parents, Drs. John and Millie Youngberg. So far, books from the series have been published into 31 languages on 6 continents. They begin with a three-volume set including, *Getting Started, Pressing Forward,* and *Finishing Strong.* These three volumes present 21 essential factors for preventing disease and enjoying optimal wellness. They expand on the foundational principles necessary for optimizing brain wellness. They are also illustrated by 1300 PowerPoint slides for small group and public presentation.[viii] *Available at winwellness.org and dryoungberg.com.*

The Bredesen Protocol Intensive with Dr. Youngberg is a 15-lecture series available for viewing on Vimeo. It includes all the lectures and discussions with Dr. Youngberg that are part of his "4-day Bredesen Protocol Intensive" designed as a clinical orientation and application of Dr. Dale Bredesen's protocol for reversing cognitive decline. This program was filmed live at the Coronado Island Marriott Resort & Spa where Dr. Youngberg periodically conducts 4-day intensives. Visit dryoungberg.co for details. Available at: *https://vimeo.com/ondemand/drwesyoungberg*

[viii] Price is $199 for the bundle pack. Available from WIN! Wellness, winwellness.org. Google *Dr. Wes Youngberg 12 Weeks to Wellness Series Highlights & Recommendations* for a series overview.

SUMMARY OF MEMORY MAKEOVER BASICS

1. Dementia is defined as a decline in mental ability severe enough to interfere with activities of daily living.
2. There are six pillars or dimensions of Alzheimer's risk. Individuals may experience one or more of these dimensions.
3. There are numerous amazing case studies indicating strategies that promote reversal of cognitive decline.
4. In Alzheimer's treatment, there is not a single drug that gives anything beyond a marginal, unsustained, symptomatic effect, with little or no effect on disease progression.
5. In order to get effective improvements in Alzheimer's, we must address the underlying causes of the disease and focus on combination strategies using a comprehensive, network-based, synergistic approach.
6. When inflammation is reduced to optimal levels, the brain has no more need to produce excess antimicrobial beta amyloid plaque, and the brain memory neurons and synapses can begin the heal.
7. The brain is like a sponge. At night during sufficient and deep sleep, it squeezes out toxic beta amyloid plaque into the spinal fluids for flushing from the body.
8. It is necessary to target multiple pathways simultaneously in order to achieve improvement in symptoms and pathophysiology.
9. The goal is not simply to normalize metabolic parameters, but rather to optimize them.
10. Just as with other chronic diseases, the objective is to reach a threshold effect—that is, to arrive at the

tipping point where the body responds to the treatment when enough of the underlying causal network components have been impacted. The pathological process can then be halted or even reversed.

11. The approach is personalized based on dozens of data points including labs, gene testing, scans, cognitive tests, and case history.

12. The protocol has continued optimization over time.

13. Healing is more likely when the factors are addressed as far upstream as possible.

14. The three goals of optimizing brain health are:

    a. **Slowing** cognitive decline. This is possible for anyone who applies the basic strategies outlined in this book.

    b. **Stopping** cognitive decline. Up to 90 percent of individuals can accomplish this.

    c. **Reversing** aspects of cognitive decline. Up to 80 percent of individuals who follow this comprehensive plan show some form of improvement in cognitive function.

15. Those who search hard for answers to their health challenges are the ones most likely to succeed.

ENDNOTES

[1] Alzheimer's Association. What is dementia? https://www.alz.org/what-is-dementia.asp. Accessed February 1, 2018.

[2] Prince MA, Emiliano; Guerchet, Maélenn; Prina, Matthew. 2014; World Alzheimer Report 2014 United Kingdom: Alzheimer's Disease International.

[3] James BD, Leurgans SE, Hebert LE, Scherr PA, Yaffe K, Bennett DA. Contribution of Alzheimer disease to mortality in the United States. *Neurology*. 2014;82:1045-1050

[4] Alzheimer's Association. 2014 Alzheimer's disease facts and figures. *Alzheimers Dement*. 2014;10:e47-e92.

[5] Public Health England. Research and analysis chapter 2: major causes of death and how they have changed. https://www. gov.uk/government/publications/health- profile-for-england/chapter-2-major-causes- of-death-and-how-they-have-changed. Published July 13, 2017. Accessed February 1, 2018.

[6] Public Health England. Research and analysis chapter 2: major causes of death and how they have changed. https://www. gov.uk/government/publications/health- profile-for-england/chapter-2-major-causes- of-death-and-how-they-have-changed. Published July 13, 2017. Accessed February 1, 2018.

[7] Bredesen DE. Reversal of cognitive decline: a novel therapeutic program. *Aging (Albany NY)*; 6(9):707–717. doi:10.18632/aging.100690

[8] Gubbels Bupp M, Jorgensen T. Androgen-Induced Immunosuppression. *Front. Immunol.*, 17 April 2018 https://doi.org/10.3389/fimmu.2018.00794

[9] Sawalha AH, Kovats S. Dehydroepiandrosterone in systemic lupus erythematosus. Curr Rheumatol Rep. 2008;10(4):286–291. doi:10.1007/s11926-008-0046-1

[10] West MJ, Gundersen HJ, J Comp Neurol. 1990 Jun 1;296(1):1-22. Unbiased stereological estimation of the number of neurons in the human hippocampus.

[11] https://www.youtube.com/watch?v=B_tjKYvEziI You can grow new brain cells. Here's how | Sandrine Thuret TED Talk Published on Oct 30, 2015

[12] Crane PK, Walker R, Hubbard RA, Li G, Nathan DM, Zheng H, et al. Glucose levels and risk of dementia. N Engl J Med. 2013;369:540–8 https://doi.org/10.1056/NEJMoa1215740.

[13] http://www.cslewisinstitute.org/The_Law_of_Undulation

[14] http://www.cslewisinstitute.org/The_Law_of_Undulation

[15] Lewis, C S. Mere Christianity. New York: Macmillan, 1960.

[16] Prov. 13: 12

[17] Schiltenwolf M, Akbar M, Hug A, Pfüller U, Gantz S, Neubauer E, Flor H, Wang H1. Evidence of specific cognitive deficits in patients with chronic low back pain under long-term substitution treatment of opioids. *Pain Physician.* 2014 Jan-Feb;17(1):9-20.

[18] Nagarkatti, Prakash et al. "Cannabinoids as novel anti-inflammatory drugs." *Future medicinal chemistry* vol. 1,7 (2009): 1333-49. doi:10.4155/fmc.09.93

[19] Iuvone, Teresa & Esposito, Giuseppe & Esposito, Ramona & Santamaria, Rita & Di Rosa, Massimo & Izzo, Angelo. (2004). Neuroprotective effect of cannabidiol, a non-psychoactive component from Cannabis sativa, on β-amyloid–induced toxicity in PC12 cells. Journal of neurochemistry. 89. 134-41.

[20] Shetty, Paulina, and Wes Youngberg. "Clinical Lifestyle Medicine Strategies for Preventing and Reversing Memory Loss in Alzheimer's." *American journal of lifestyle medicine* vol. 12,5 391-395. 11 May. 2018, doi:10.1177/1559827618766468

[21] Baker S. *Detoxification and healing: the key to optimal health.* New York, NY: McGraw-Hill; 2003.

[22] Baker S. *Detoxification and healing: the key to optimal health.* New York, NY: McGraw-Hill; 2003.

[23] Bredesen DE, Amos EC, Canick J, et al. Reversal of cognitive decline in Alzheimer's disease. *Aging (Albany NY).* 2016;8:1250- 1258.

[24] Cousins N. *Anatomy of an Illness: As Perceived by the Patient.* New York, NY: W W Norton; 2005.

[25] Bredesen DE. Reversal of cognitive decline: a novel therapeutic program. *Aging* (Albany NY). 2014;6:707-717.

[26] Vivian Teichberg, and Luba Vikhanski, Protecting the Brain from a Glutamate Storm. Cerebrum May 10, 2007. http://www.dana.org/Cerebrum/2007/Protecting_the_Brain_from_a_Glutamate_Storm/

[27] Lewerenz J, Maher P. Chronic Glutamate Toxicity in Neurodegenerative Diseases-What is the Evidence?. Front Neurosci. 2015;9:469. Published 2015 Dec 16. doi:10.3389/fnins.2015.00469

[28] Association of homocysteine with hippocampal volume independent of cerebral amyloid and vascular burden. Choe Y.M., Sohn B.K., Choi H.J., Byun M.S., Seo E.H., Han J.Y., Kim Y.K., (...), Lee D.Y. (2014) *Neurobiology of Aging*, 35 (7) , pp. 1519-1525.

[29] Herrmann, W. & Obeid, R. (2011). Homocysteine: a biomarker in neurodegenerative diseases. *Clinical Chemistry and Laboratory Medicine*, 49(3), pp. 435-441. Retrieved 1 Apr. 2019, from doi:10.1515/CCLM.2011.084

[30] Ma, Fei, Tianfeng Wu, Jiangang Zhao, Lu Ji, Aili Song, Meilin Zhang and Guowei Huang. "Plasma Homocysteine and Serum Folate and Vitamin B12 Levels in Mild Cognitive Impairment and Alzheimer's Disease: A Case-Control Study." *Nutrients*(2017).

[31] A. Vogiatzoglou, H. Refsum, C. Johnston, S.M. Smith, K.M. Bradle, C. de Jager, M.M. Budge, A.D. Smith. Vitamin B12 status and rate of brain volume loss in community-dwelling elderly. Neurology, 71 (2008), pp. 826-832

[32] Williams JH, Pereira EA, Budge MM, Bradley KM. Minimal hippocampal width relates to plasma homocysteine in community-dwelling older people. Age Ageing. 2002;31:440–444.

[33] Celeste A. de Jager, Critical levels of brain atrophy associated with homocysteine and cognitive decline, Neurobiology of Aging, Volume 35, Supplement 2, 2014, Pages S35-S39, ISSN 0197-4580

[34] Bredesen DE. Metabolic profiling distinguishes three subtypes of Alzheimer's disease. *Aging (Albany NY)*. 2015;7: 595-600.

[35] Bredesen D. The end of Alzheimer's: the first program to prevent and reverse cognitive decline. New York, NY: Penguin Random House, 2017.

[36] Bredesen DE. Reversal of cognitive decline: a novel therapeutic program. *Aging* (Albany NY). 2014;6:707-717.

[37] A.Vogiatzoglou, H. Refsum, C. Johnston, S.M. Smith, K.M. Bradley, C. de Jager, M.M. Budge, A.D. Smith. Vitamin B12 status and rate of brain volume loss in community-dwelling elderly. Neurology, 71 (2008), pp. 826-832

[38] Burns JM, Johnson DK, Watts A, Swerdlow RH, Brooks WM Reduced lean mass in early Alzheimer disease and its association with brain atrophy.
Arch Neurol. 2010 Apr; 67(4):428-33.

[39] Mandsager K, Harb S, Cremer P, Phelan D, Nissen SE, Jaber W. Association of Cardiorespiratory Fitness With Long-term Mortality Among Adults Undergoing Exercise Treadmill Testing. *JAMA Netw Open.* Published online October 19, 20181(6):e183605. doi:10.1001/jamanetworkopen.2018.3605.

[40] Abbayya, Keshava et al. "Association between Periodontitis and Alzheimer's Disease." *North American journal of medical sciences* vol. 7,6 (2015): 241-6. doi:10.4103/1947-2714.159325

[41] Tan ZS, Beiser A, Vasan RS, et al. Thyroid function and the risk of Alzheimer disease: the Framingham Study. *Arch Intern Med.* 2008;168(14):1514–1520. doi:10.1001/archinte.168.14.1514

[42] https://www.lifeextension.com/Magazine/2007/11/report_pregnen olone/Page-01

[43] Schumacher M, Weill-Engerer S, Liere P, et al. Steroid hormones and neurosteroids in normal and pathological aging of the nervous system. Prog Neurobiol. 2003 Sep;71(1):3-29.

[44] Manzanero S, Erion JR, Santro T, et al. Intermittent fasting attenuates increases in neurogenesis after ischemia and reperfusion and improves recovery. *J Cereb Blood Flow Metab.* 2014;34(5):897–905. doi:10.1038/jcbfm.2014.36

[45] Anton SD, Moehl K, Donahoo WT, et al. Flipping the Metabolic Switch: Understanding and Applying the Health Benefits of Fasting. *Obesity (Silver Spring).* 2018;26(2):254–268. doi:10.1002/oby.22065

[46] Benjamin JS, Pilarowski GO, Carosso GA, et al. A ketogenic diet rescues hippocampal memory defects in a mouse model of Kabuki syndrome. *Proc Natl Acad Sci U S A.* 2017;114(1):125–130. doi:10.1073/pnas.1611431114

[47] Bredesen DE. Reversal of cognitive decline: a novel therapeutic program. *Aging* (Albany NY). 2014;6:707-717.

[48] Page 19 in: Stephen K. Bangert MA MB BChir MSc MBA FRCPath; William J. Marshall MA MSc MBBS FRCP FRCPath FRCPEdin FIBiol; Marshall, William Leonard (2008). Clinical biochemistry: metabolic and clinical aspects. Philadelphia: Churchill Livingstone/Elsevier. ISBN 978-0-443-10186-1.

[49] Circulation. Heart Disease and Stroke Statistics—2019 Update: A Report From the American Heart Association March 5, 2019 - Volume 139, Issue 10

[50] Brewer GJ. Alzheimer's disease causation by copper toxicity and treatment with zinc. Front Aging Neurosci. 2014;6:92. Published 2014 May 16. doi:10.3389/fnagi.2014.00092

[51] Avan A., Hoogenraad T.U. Zinc and Copper in Alzheimer's Disease. JAD. 2015;46:89–92. doi: 10.3233/JAD-150186.

[52] www.sungenomics.com taken from Internet, May 3, 2019.

[53] https://www.hopkinsmedicine.org/news/articles/researchers-discover-death-and-rebirth-of-the-gut-brain as of 6/10/19

[54] Secades, Julio. (2019). Citicoline in the Treatment of Cognitive Impairment. Journal of Neurology & Experimental Neuroscience. 5(1): 14-26. 10.17756/jnen.2019-047.

[55] Farooqui AA, Farooqui T, Madan A, Ong JH, Ong WY. Ayurvedic Medicine for the Treatment of Dementia: Mechanistic Aspects. *Evid Based Complement Alternat Med.* 2018;2018:2481076. Published 2018 May 15. doi:10.1155/2018/2481076

[56] Rao RV, Descamps O, John V, Bredesen DE. Ayurvedic medicinal plants for Alzheimer's disease: a review. *Alzheimers Res Ther.* 2012;4(3):22. Published 2012 Jun 29. doi:10.1186/alzrt125

[57] Christine Barba, One Day There Will Be a Treatment for Alzheimer's. Until Then, Follow This Advice. *Being Patient: The latest news on Alzheimer's disease and brain health research.* August 2, 2018. https://www.beingpatient.com/alzheimers-prevention-2/

[58] Sehgal N, Gupta A, Valli RK, et al. Withania somnifera reverses Alzheimer's disease pathology by enhancing low-density lipoprotein receptor-related protein in liver. *Proc Natl Acad Sci U S A.* 2012;109(9):3510–3515. doi:10.1073/pnas.1112209109

[59] Chen M, Du ZY, Zheng X, Li DL, Zhou RP, Zhang K. Use of curcumin in diagnosis, prevention, and treatment of Alzheimer's disease. *Neural Regen Res.* 2018;13(4):742–752. doi:10.4103/1673-5374.230303

[60] Calabrese C, Gregory WL, Leo M, Kraemer D, Bone K, Oken B. Effects of a standardized Bacopa monnieri extract on cognitive performance, anxiety, and depression in the elderly: a randomized, double-blind, placebo-controlled trial. *J Altern Complement Med.* 2008;14(6):707–713. doi:10.1089/acm.2008.0018

[61] Bacopa: A powerful herb to improve memory and brain health. Dena Schmidt, staff writer. NaturalHealth365, January 8, 2017. https://www.naturalhealth365.com/bacopa-brain-health-2096.html

[62] Roodenrys S[1], Booth D, Bulzomi S, Phipps A, Micallef C, Smoker J. Chronic effects of Brahmi (Bacopa monnieri) on human memory. Neuropsychopharmacology. 2002 Aug;27(2):279-81.

[63] Con Stough, Hemant Singh, and Andrea Zangara, "Mechanisms, Efficacy, and Safety of Bacopa monnieri(Brahmi) for Cognitive and Brain Enhancement," Evidence-Based Complementary and Alternative Medicine, vol. 2015, Article ID 717605, 2 pages, 2015. https://doi.org/10.1155/2015/717605.

[64] https://www.drweil.com/health-wellness/balanced-living/meet-dr-weil/about-andrew-weil-m-d/

[65] http://beclifelonglearner.blogspot.com/2009/05/insights-into-cs-lewis-his-mothers.html

[66] Dale E Bredesen, Kenneth Sharlin, David Jenkins, Miki Okuno, Wes Youngberg, Sharon Hausman Cohen, Anne Stefani, Ronald L Brown, Seth Conger, Craig Tanio, Ann Hathaway, Mikhail Kogan, David Hagedorn, Edwin Amos, Amylee Amos, Nathaniel Bergman, Carol Diamond, Jean Lawrence, Ilene Naomi Rusk, Patricia Henry and Mary Braud. Reversal of Cognitive Decline: 100 Patients. *Journal of Alzheimer's Disease & Parkinsonism.* 2018, 8:5.